The Smile of Your Dreams

The Smile of Your Dreams

Birmingham Orthodontics' Guide to an Exceptional Patient Experience

Michael McCarthy, DMD

Erika Hartman, DDS

Careybeth Rivers, DMD, MS

Published by Advantage, Charleston, South Carolina.
Member of Advantage Media Group.

ADVANTAGE is a registered trademark, and the Advantage colophon is a trademark of Advantage Media Group, Inc.

Printed in the United States of America.

10 9 8 7 6 5 4 3 2 1

ISBN: 978-1-64225-030-5
LCCN: 2018937710

This publication is designed to provide accurate and authoritative information in regard to the subject matter covered. It is sold with the understanding that the publisher is not engaged in rendering legal, accounting, or other professional services. If legal advice or other expert assistance is required, the services of a competent professional person should be sought.

Advantage Media Group is proud to be a part of the Tree Neutral® program. Tree Neutral offsets the number of trees consumed in the production and printing of this book by taking proactive steps such as planting trees in direct proportion to the number of trees used to print books. To learn more about Tree Neutral, please visit **www.treeneutral.com**.

Advantage Media Group is a publisher of business, self-improvement, and professional development books. We help entrepreneurs, business leaders, and professionals share their Stories, Passion, and Knowledge to help others Learn & Grow. Do you have a manuscript or book idea that you would like us to consider for publishing? Please visit **advantagefamily.com** or call **1.866.775.1696**.

TABLE OF CONTENTS

FOREWORD: FROM THE FOUNDER OF BIRMINGHAM ORTHODONTICS. XI

INTRODUCTION:. 1

CHAPTER ONE: WHY IS MY CHILD'S SMILE SO IMPORTANT?. 17

CHAPTER TWO: WHY DO KIDS NEED BRACES?. 25

CHAPTER THREE: WHY NOT JUST A DENTIST? WHY AN ORTHODONTIST? 31

CHAPTER FOUR: CHOOSE A HIGHLY SUCCESSFUL ORTHODONTIST. 39

CHAPTER FIVE: WHAT CAN I EXPECT AT THE INITIAL CONSULTATION AND EXAM?. 49

CHAPTER SIX: SHOULDN'T THERE BE A GUARANTEE? . . 55

CHAPTER SEVEN: HOW TO GET MORE INFORMATION. . 59

CHAPTER EIGHT: HOW TO PAY FOR ORTHODONTIC TREATMENT AND BRACES 63

CHAPTER NINE: WHAT ARE THE TREATMENT OPTIONS?. 77

CHAPTER TEN: HOW DIFFICULT IS LIVING WITH BRACES 91

CHAPTER ELEVEN: LIFE AFTER BRACES: RETAINERS . . .101

CHAPTER TWELVE: LET'S CELEBRATE!. 105

CHAPTER THIRTEEN: WHAT ABOUT MY SMILE?. 109

FAQ 113

RESOURCES 123

ABOUT THE AUTHORS 125

THE NEXT STEP 128

YOUR CUSTOMIZED SMILE ANALYSIS 129

Foreword

From the Founder of Birmingham Orthodontics

My name is Dr. Michael McCarthy. I'm an orthodontist and the founder of Birmingham Orthodontics. My reasons for becoming an orthodontist and forming an organization for exceptionally successful orthodontists leading the field in both clinical and patient care—instead of becoming a veterinarian or handsome movie actor or professor of poetry—are easily found in another section of this book, if you're curious. They might matter to you.

But this book is about *you,* the parent, and your son or daughter, not about me. It's about information you need to know to make intelligent, responsible decisions about your child's health, appearance, self-esteem, and social interactions ... of a permanent, lifelong nature. Does your child really *need* braces? If so, when? If so, who should you trust to provide his orthodontic care? How will you know you're not being ripped off?

This book isn't *Fifty Shades of Gray*. It just can't be that exciting. But if you take the time to read this book, you'll know how to confidently and correctly make whatever decisions you need to make about your child's orthodontic care.

It's *not* 1982.

To start, we're no longer dealing with heavy, ugly, tight, painful metal braces—every visit to have them tightened was another round of torture; they were hard to put on, hard to keep on, painful to remove, and it was irritating having a list of foods and activities to avoid for a long period of time. If your child needs braces now, the experience won't be anything like it was when you were a kid. He won't even try hiding under the bed and have to be dragged kicking and screaming to the car to visit my office.

Not only has *everything* about braces changed, but now all braces are created differently. So try to get that horrible, metal-mouth image out of your head. You're probably aware of invisible braces, maybe by a brand name: Invisalign. That's what prompts a lot of patients to call or email me in the first place. However, Invisalign is but one of a number of options to be considered to get to *the* best, customized, and personalized answer to your child's needs. You don't want to equate this to buying something over the counter: "Hey, give me Invisalign. How much?" It's more complicated than that. But it's a good representation of modern braces. They can be (nearly) invisible, pliable and with lighter steel, safer, and even self-removable for hygiene or sports and easily put back in place. They're not painful and achieve more certain results in a shorter period of time.

When I was growing up, a lot of kids didn't get braces they really needed and their parents let them off the hook, either because they believed their child couldn't tolerate the pain or because the cost was just beyond the family's budget. Now that braces are virtually painless, what about the cost?

Today's far better braces cost *less* than the one-size-damn-well-will-fit-all, metal-mouth braces of the '60s, '70s, and '80s. They cost as little as one Starbucks drink a day for a year, rarely more than twice that, and there are a number of different payment plans available if needed. So, that second hurdle is a lot lower than it was when our parents encountered it.

In other words, the first of my two introductory messages is: *relax.*

I've got your back. It's going to be okay—better than okay, easier than okay, and more convenient than okay. Orthodontic procedures *won't* hurt your child, and he or she will surprise you by not complaining it does. It's *not* going to hurt your bank account; you won't be reduced to a backyard stay-cation next summer and the summer after that. It's *not* going to be a maddening maelstrom of appointments of uncertain length, or hours in a waiting room. Not at *my* office.

More Than Just Braces

My second introductory message is: this is about more than just braces.

Orthodontic care for a child, preteen, teen and even an adult is more than just correcting crooked, crowded teeth with braces. That's like thinking diabetes only needs attention when feet have to be amputated, or getting tires checked might be a good idea after being stranded with a flat at night while it's pouring rain.

"Thank you for making our experience with braces pleasant and happy. As a busy working mom, I never knew it would be this easy and affordable."

—MARIA R.

xiv • MCCARTHY • HARTMAN • RIVERS

Orthodontic checkups *by an orthodontist*[1], starting at age eight or nine, are a proper part of child rearing. In many cases, prevention is less troublesome and less costly. Even if you're late getting your son or daughter in, it's still possible they won't need braces and that other treatment options will do. But if they do need braces, the sooner you know of the options, the better.

This is also about more than just braces because it impacts psychological and emotional health, not just oral health. This is discussed later in the book.

Why It's Important

1. Straight teeth function better, are easier to clean, and are more likely to last a lifetime.

2. People with straight, well-aligned teeth can avoid gum disease, which has very serious health ramifications.

3. Properly aligned jaws reduce the risk of temporomandibular joint disorders (TMJ), which can ruin sleep or cause chronic headaches or migraines.

4. Both kids and adults with great smiles feel better about themselves, and that can greatly increase their confidence.

Some parents put off orthodontic treatment, but these irregularities and problems do *not* heal themselves. *This isn't acne; they don't grow out of it.* The problems only grow worse and harder to resolve with age.

---

1   All orthodontists are dentists, but dentists are *not* the same as or suitable substitutes for orthodontists. Read on to find out more.

Don't Ask Them to Hide Their Smile

Never smiling isn't easy in an age of selfies and social media. Children can become self-conscious—painfully self-conscious—and embarrassed. "No thanks, Mom, I'd rather just stay home."

Teen suicide has skyrocketed since social media shaming and bullying rose to ugly prominence. Teen depression affects everything from getting the good grades needed to get into a good college to first dates, first loves, and enjoying (or hating) their childhood and teen years. But it doesn't stop there. Uncorrected, bad smiles go with them to college and into their career.

This isn't just cosmetic either. It's also medical and can be a serious detriment to their health.

So, read on. Be informed. Be able to ask smart questions and do the right thing. I guarantee you'll be much better able to correctly and confidently make good choices for your family through this book.

Michael McCarthy, DMD
Founder, Birmingham Orthodontics
Diplomate, American Board of Orthodontics

Introduction

WHAT MAKES BIRMINGHAM Orthodontics unique? We can point to many things we're proud of: our twenty-five years in business and the more than twenty-five thousand patients we've treated; the 2017 *Birmingham's Best Small Business* award we received from the Birmingham Business Journal; the fact that some of our patients love us so much they're willing to drive long distances to get to us—up to four hours each way! But we believe our success is based on our shared dedication to our mission: to provide exceptional orthodontic care at an affordable price, and to transform the lives and the smiles of our patients, our staff, and our community. That's what has kept us inspired every day—since day one.

That mission was what motivated Dr. Michael McCarthy to create Birmingham Orthodontics. While serving as a dentist and a Green Beret in the U.S. Army, Dr. McCarthy could see that his daughter was going to need braces. But when he sought orthodontic treatment for her, he realized for the first time how expensive it was, and that paying for it would be a challenge on a military family's budget. That inspired Dr. McCarthy to become an orthodontist dedicated to providing the best possible care, while keeping the price affordable.

After serving in the Army for ten years, Dr. McCarthy decided to make his home in Birmingham, Alabama and he opened his first offices in that area in 1993. Today, Birmingham Orthodontics has four locations and is the leader in making first-class orthodontic treatment affordable. Dr. McCarthy went against the prevailing practice of charging patients $1000–$2000 or more to get started in braces, and instead, offered all patients the financial option of getting started in braces with no initial down payment and low monthly fees for treatment. That has put orthodontics within reach of many families in the area who otherwise could not have afforded the help they needed. We understand. Our patient families work hard and these days it seems like everything is expensive, especially when you have kids. But it's our philosophy that orthodontics shouldn't just be available for the few.

In many areas in life, a lower cost comes with lower quality, but that's not true in our practice. Instead, we work more efficiently so we can provide excellent care while keeping costs down for our patients. How good are we? Birmingham Orthodontics participated in a unique study to evaluate the quality of orthodontic treatment received. In the study, the orthodontists presented their patient records at the beginning and at the end of treatment. The records were measured and evaluated for the quality of treatment and compared to other orthodontists who were chosen to be the comparison standards based on their reputation, experience, and credentials. It was tough for the study's author to find participants, because doctors aren't usually eager to open themselves up for criticism. But Dr. McCarthy was happy to share our results with the researchers. He felt that if the practice did well in the study, then that would be great—and if not, then the information we'd get could help us improve patient outcomes.

But our results were excellent. Overall, the findings of the study showed that Birmingham Orthodontics treated orthodontic cases that were more severe at the beginning of treatment and were able to provide the same high quality of care as the comparison practices.[2] We treat all kinds of patients, from all walks of life—and all with the same high standard of care and respect for the patient's needs.

In 2004, Dr. McCarthy was very fortunate to be joined by Dr. Erika Hartman. Dr. Hartman is an excellent orthodontist and a very compassionate person who quickly developed relationships with both the patients and staff to enhance the mission of Birmingham Orthodontics. She is very caring and this is reflected in the love that our patients have for her. Dr. Hartman graduated from Meharry Medical College where one of the missions there is to educate doctors that will serve the underserved. With that mission in mind, she was intrigued with Birmingham Orthodontics' philosophy of providing quality orthodontic care at an affordable price. She joined the team and has loved being able to provide great care to so many people who would normally not have been able to afford braces.

With the addition of Dr. Hartman, we were able to better serve our patients by expanding our office hours and making appointments more available to our patient's needs. In addition, we were

---

2   Donald R. Poulton, Sheldon Baumrind, and Vicki Vlaskalic, "Treatment outcomes in 3 modes of orthodontic practice," *American Journal of Orthodontics and Dentofacial Orthopedics* 121, no. 2 (February 2002): 176–184, https://doi. org/10.1067/mod.2002.121640

able to open a third location in Alabaster which made travel more convenient for our patients.

Patients love Birmingham Orthodontics and the practice has continued to grow in response to its mission and to the care its patients have received. In fact, the response has been so tremendous that by 2012, Birmingham Orthodontics was in need of another orthodontist to help meet the patient demand. We were very fortunate to be joined by Dr. Careybeth Rivers, who was also attracted to our mission of providing exceptional orthodontic care at an affordable price, and transforming the lives and the smiles of our patients, our staff, and our community. Dr. Rivers is an excellent orthodontist and works exceptionally hard at keeping costs in check so we can continue to provide the best of care at prices families can afford. This is very rare in medicine today and we are proud to continue to be leaders in providing this to our patients. She also has developed excellent relationships with both patients and staff. Dr. Rivers is involved with several charities in Birmingham and has helped expand Birmingham Orthodontics' participation in charitable organizations.

The success of Birmingham Orthodontics continues to attract new patients every day. This in turn has allowed us to expand our staff and put systems in place to better serve our patients and their needs, as well as giving us the good fortune of adding more fantastic doctors to our staff. In 2016, we were fortunate to have Dr. Katelyn Feinberg and Dr. Andrew Havron become members of our orthodontic family. We also opened a fourth location in Greystone which makes our offices and appointment times even more convenient for our patients.

All of our orthodontists have received their orthodontic education from some of the finest institutions in the country, including the University of Alabama School of Dentistry, Howard University, and the University of Michigan. These programs all provide exceptional educational experiences, and having this kind of diversity of education and experience is an important factor in the quality of treatment we offer. Why? Because in orthodontics, you can go to three different doctors and have three different treatment plans. Some complex cases present particular difficulties and having this wealth of knowledge and diversity of experience from these different institutions under one roof means that our doctors can always get a second opinion from a colleague when they need it. That's especially critical when we're looking at cases that involve facial surgeries or for adults that are getting their teeth set up for crown and bridge, replacement of teeth, or implants. We each take on cases like that; and while it's important that you have the continuity of care throughout the different parts of treatment, we do check and double-check each other's work, because five heads are better than one. If you're a single practitioner, you don't have the luxury of colleagues on hand to offer their input.

And having five doctors on staff also makes it easier for you to get an appointment with one of them at a time most convenient for you.

We Value Your Time As Much As You Do

We understand that nothing is more frustrating than showing up on time for a doctor's appointment and having to wait all day in the waiting room. That's why we get you in for treatment on time so you can get on with your day. And you won't feel rushed; we've got a big enough staff to ensure that if your case demands a little more attention, you'll get the time you need. For us, the most important person in the office is always the person in the chair. That's not always the case in other practices; there's another orthodontist we know of who opened his office up on Saturdays but doesn't take appointments, which means his patients have to wait, sometimes for hours, to be seen. Not surprisingly, a lot of those patients leave his care and come to us.

Other practices make you come back multiple times after your initial assessment to take care of things like getting records done, or to have your braces put on. We don't. Once you've gotten your initial examination and your assessment with the doctor, all the details are dealt with then and there. The majority of cases don't require extractions, so if braces need to go on, we place them that same day, so there's no need to make multiple appointments. We pioneered this "quick start" process in our area, and our patients really appreciate it.

Our doctors and our office staff never stop learning, and we're proud to offer the latest technology and advances in care. That means your time in treatment will be more comfortable and, in many cases, briefer. And the intervals between your office visits will be longer too, meaning fewer appointments for you and less disruption of your busy day.

We Never Stop Improving Your Experience

Too often great customer service gets talked about, but falls between the cracks in practice, because the doctors running the office aren't willing to make the ongoing investment in staffing and services required to keep up with their patients' needs. At Birmingham Orthodontics, our office operations are constantly being refined and upgraded to ensure that our patients' experiences are uniformly excellent, and to ultimately fine-tune our processes.

We firmly believe that our doctors should be seeing patients and not be tasked with running the business aspects of the practice, because that's not what they're here for. Our receptionists should be greeting and taking care of you as soon as you walk through our doors. Birmingham Orthodontics takes special care in running the practice "behind the scenes" so our patients can get the best service whether they are in the office, on the phone, or online.

To help provide enhanced customer service, we have brought on a CEO to run and to manage the business aspects of the practice, because our doctors need to be free to focus their time and energy treating patients. Because your time and convenience are of utmost importance to us, Birmingham Orthodontics has hired an experienced, full-time trainer to continually improve our customer care and services. She sits with the front-desk staff to teach them how to work better with patients; she works with the treatment coordinators, helping them serve you better when your plan for treatment is being finalized. She assists us in managing the flow of patients through the office more efficiently so everyone's comfortable and nobody has to wait for their appointment. Our office has even taken our commitment to great customer service one step further. We encourage all of our patients to provide feedback after their visit, especially if they find anything about our services lacking in any area so we can address it at our next staff training. At the beginning of each month, we shut down our entire company for half a day to better train our staff on how they can better serve our patients.

And we don't stop there; we regularly send our staff outside of the office for seminars on service and how to improve it. Next year, we are planning to work with Ritz Carlton and the Disney Institute—recognized as two of the finest service training organizations in the world—to provide even better support to our patients.

Have you ever gone into a professional office on time for your appointment, only to be left to cool your heels while the receptionist at the desk talks to someone else on the phone? We have, and we find it unacceptable. That's why Birmingham Orthodontics is the leader in establishing a call center for our patients. We made the decision a long time ago to take the telephones away from the front receptionist desks in our offices. Our call center is staffed by members of our front office personnel rather than having calls be outsourced to another company. By having our personnel not having to answer phones while working at the front desk, we can be more attentive to our patient needs when they come in to our offices. By having our front office personnel also staff the call center, we can assure that all callers are taken care of by someone familiar with them and the practice. This may seem like a small detail, but it has made a profound difference in our service to our patients.

Our care and attention to details like that are why our patients often go to great lengths to be in our practice—literally. We have patients who travel from other states such as Tennessee, Georgia, Florida, and Mississippi just to see us. Recently, a mother of a former patient's called us; she lives in northern Alabama and has a daughter in need of treatment. We scheduled an appointment to see her daughter, and if she's ready to get started, we will place braces the same day and help schedule appointments, since she has a long way to drive and we want to maximize treatment for each appointment. And this story isn't unique; whole families pass through our practice, from the youngest member to Mom and Dad.

Why a Great Smile Matters

Orthodontic treatment can change lives. Having a great smile inspires confidence in yourself and in your appearance. It has a critical effect on how you're perceived by others, too—as smarter, more attractive, more successful, and more confident. And a great smile (or a bad one) will likely impact your success in life, as well as your personal happiness. Throughout this book, you will see many examples of how a bad smile and bite can negatively impact your life.

In our view, orthodontic treatment is one of the greatest investments you can ever make, whether for yourself or your child. When weighing the costs of orthodontics, consider what not having them may cost you or you child in terms of lifelong happiness and success.

We're always glad to see our former patients when they come back for a visit. A young man who'd needed extensive work when he was a child dropped by recently to share the news that he'd gotten a track scholarship at the University of Miami. He'd come so far from the quiet and withdrawn child he'd been when we first met him. He's completely changed—he feels great about himself. He's a big time athlete in his circle, and he has a lot of big plans for the future. And his isn't an unusual story; so many children excel when they come out of their shells and start to feel good about themselves.

The Problem of Bullying

Almost every day we have kids coming into our office who are suffering from teasing and bullying from their peers at school because of their appearance. It's heartbreaking to see how these kids will hang their heads, cover their mouths when they speak, or simply not speak at all because they're ashamed of how they look. That kind of start in life leaves scars. And a child who won't speak up in class or interact with others may be seen as slow or antisocial, when the problem is really just low self-esteem.

That's why we offer early orthodontic treatment care for those who need it. All children should be evaluated for orthodontic care by age seven or eight. Sometimes this evaluation is done by the pediatric dentist or by your general dentist, and other times it is done by the orthodontist—but you don't need to wait for a referral, and you certainly shouldn't wait for the child's permanent teeth to come in if you see a problem. While many children may benefit from braces at an early age, not all of them need early treatment, and we will give you an honest assessment.

We look for problems such as crossbites, excessive crowding/ spacing, bad habits, and social/self-esteem issues that will have a negative effect if not treated immediately. For these cases, we will recommend treatment with the understanding that full orthodontic treatment will probably be needed when the child is older. For those not having major early treatment issues, we will advise them that we can wait on orthodontic treatment until the child is older. Most cases fall into this category, but for those that don't, early intervention can be crucial.

When kids who have been bullied come in to get their braces, we can see their attitude change almost immediately. They leave that initial appointment already feeling a little better about themselves, because they know they're on the road to improvement. And when the real improvements start to show, the cloud of shyness that hung over them when they first came to us lifts, and we see the exuberant, sociable child that had been hidden underneath it. Sometimes when those braces come off, there are tears—happy tears—from Mom, and many times there are hugs all around and heartfelt thank yous. We never get tired of seeing those kinds of transformations or of hearing, "You changed my life!"

And It's Not Just for Kids

Are you ashamed of your smile? If you are, you probably know what it's like to be that person who reflexively turns their head away when they laugh or when they're in a group picture. There are so many ways that people cover up what embarrasses them. Some people even lose their smiles, permanently—and a smile's a terrible thing to lose. But today, more and more adults are opting to get the smiles they've always wanted. So many of our adult patients have sacrificed their needs for their children's, making sure they were taken care of first. Many of them have children who were patients in our practice. Now that the kids are grown, the moms and dads are coming in, telling us, "It's my turn—I'm ready to spend some time and some money on myself, and make myself look better and feel better."

And with the many new options in treatment that you'll learn about as you read this book, that treatment can often be invisible, or nearly so—you don't need to feel self-conscious about being seen in braces. Often, the adults that come to see us for orthodontics make the choice because of a change in their lives. Maybe they're back in the dating scene or are hoping for a promotion at work and know how much their personal appearance matters as they move up the ladder.

Whatever your reason, don't wait another day to get the smile you've always wanted. It's faster, easier, and more affordable than you might think—and your consultation is always free.

We Care About the Community

We're grateful to be a valued presence here in Alabama, and we do our best to give back to the community we call home. We were the very first provider in the state to sign on with the national organization Smiles Change Lives, which provides free orthodontic treatment to children whose families couldn't otherwise afford them. We've happily taken on every case they've sent us, providing the same standard of care for these children as we do for all our patients. It's a great organization and we're proud to have been a part of it for many years.

Before that, we worked with local churches to provide braces for low or no cost to needy members of their communities. And we often donate the costs of our services as a raffle item to schools or churches trying to raise money.

One of the more innovative ways we encourage our staff to get engaged in local charities is that we pay our staff members for the time they spend working at different charitable organizations. We choose about five of these charities each year, places like the Ronald McDonald house or local animal shelters, and the staff member goes to work there for a day. Sometimes at the holidays, they'll go work at a local homeless shelter or food bank. It's great for the staff because they get to pitch in and help these great organizations, without having to carve out the time to do it away from work or having to give up their income. We're glad to support their efforts and give back in this way.

Why Choose Birmingham Orthodontics?

We firmly believe we're your best choice—but you don't have to take our word for it. Birmingham Orthodontics has a five-star rating and has received over five hundred five-star ratings on both Google and Facebook. Our CEO, Brian McCarthy, was a finalist for Birmingham's Top CEO and was listed as one of Birmingham's top "40 Under 40" business leaders by the *Birmingham Business Journal*. In both 2017 and 2018 Birmingham Orthodontics was voted "Best Orthodonist" by *Birmingham Magazine* and has been named as either Favorite Orthodontist or runner-up to Favorite Orthodontist over twenty times in various local magazines and newspapers.

Many of our employees are either our former patients or parents of former patients. Our patients' reviews speak volumes, not just about our stellar results and the level of care they receive from our doctors and technicians, but also about how they're treated—like valued family and friends. We respect our patients, and that shows in every interaction we have, from your first phone call to the day you get your retainer.

We are the leaders in orthodontic practice marketing and patient education. Since 1993, we have been educating the community on the importance, affordability, ease, and benefits of orthodontic treatment. We have strived to increase awareness of the importance of general dental treatment too, not just orthodontic care. We advise parents on the proper timing of orthodontic care for their children and do not just place braces on their teeth because they showed up that day. We provide help in developing treatment plans for patients requiring all manners of comprehensive dental treatment, including children's dentistry, full mouth reconstruction, replacement of missing teeth with dental implants and crowns and bridges, periodontal and gum disease, and corrective jaw surgery.

The most important thing, of course, is the quality of care you'll receive here, where we are second to none. Experience counts when it comes to medicine, and what really matters is how many times the doctor has done a procedure. At Birmingham Orthodontics, we have treated over twenty-five thousand patients and have done so with exceptionally high service ratings. Our orthodontists have been recognized with prestigious awards such as being named as one of "America's Top Dentists." Others have been published in leading orthodontic journals and have received Board Certification Status by the American Board of Orthodontics.

Affordability is a big part of our mission, because we believe you shouldn't have to go deep into debt to pay for orthodontics. Our straightforward pricing policies make it easy for you to get the care you need for yourself or your child. No down payment, low monthly payments, 0 percent interest financing—this puts orthodontic treatment within reach for many families that might otherwise not be able to afford it and puts money back in the pockets of those who can. You should never choose your practitioner based solely on cost, of course—but with the great service, convenience, and quality of care provided by Birmingham Orthodontics, why pay more?

And we're conveniently close to where you are. Birmingham Orthodontics has four offices located near major highways and is open five days a week. There is always an office and a doctor available on these days, so you've got no worries if your regular doctor is on vacation, because we have you covered.

Why choose us? Because quality of care, customer service, and affordability are important to you; they're important to all of us at Birmingham Orthodontics, too. Give us a call.

Chapter One

Why Is My Child's Smile So Important?

IF YOU ARE WEIGHING the yes/no and now/later decisions of orthodontic care or braces, you'll be trying to decide just how important or unimportant it really is.

Some parents feel "looks aren't everything." Some think their kid should just be tough-minded about this and not overly sensitive. Some may not have had orthodontic care when they were children and think, *Hey, I turned out just fine. I have a great spouse, a good career, friends—so what's the big deal?*

But that was then. This is *now*: the age of social media.

Social shaming and bullying is a lot worse, a lot more common, and a lot more persistent than when you were a kid. Teen suicide is on the rise, and such suicides share one thing in common: shocked and bewildered parents who could not conceive of their child ending his own life. Sure, they might've noticed he was a *little* depressed. They knew he was being bullied and spending more time home, alone, not leaving his room, but geez, he *is* a teenager, after all. What once were a few days or weeks of misery contained in the cafeteria with a few bullies is now endless, expansive, and broadcast online to everybody. Behind a computer screen, it can get far nastier than most would dare in person. Sometimes, kids bully each other for no reason, being a buck-toothed girl or a boy with gaps in between their teeth is enough to exacerbate the situation.

Signs Your Child May Be Being Bullied

- decrease in self-esteem
- not wanting to go to school skipping school
- injuries they can't explain
- self-destructive behaviors (e.g., harming themselves)
- declining school grades
- sleep difficulties
- loss of interest in schoolwork or activities
- sudden loss of friends or avoiding social groups
- changes in eating habits

A straight, clean and healthy smile can not only give your child the confidence she needs to embrace her true worth, but can also pave the way toward easier socialization at school, church, or during extracurricular activities. Do your child a favor and talk about her smile and how it might be affecting her.

Beyond that, there's a life ahead of your child. Going to junior high with crooked teeth and a humiliating smile is one thing. Hey, plenty of kids are going to school *without shoes* for heaven's sake. But going to college admission interviews, packing up and heading off to college, going to job interviews, trying to fit into new and anxiety-rich environments at a faraway college or new workplace with a bad smile—and maybe unavoidable bad breath with it—and daytime headaches from nighttime teeth-grinding is a lot more serious.

This isn't *just* a cosmetic issue. Misaligned, crooked teeth equal *significant* medical problems.

Poorly aligned teeth can produce chronic headaches and migraines, contribute to digestive problems because of the inability to properly chew foods, and make getting a decent night's sleep impossible. Perhaps the most dangerous of all: it can foster gum disease. Gum disease has absolute links to diabetes, heart disease, strokes and dementia, as well as, of course, the loss of natural teeth altogether. While getting braces as an adult is still an option, the process is much easier and less painful if orthodontic corrections are made as a child.

Uncorrected mouth problems and misaligned teeth make for strangely stretched gums inevitably destined to separate from teeth. This could allow "pockets" for infections and periodontal disease to arise and turn into *very* difficult, painful, and costly problems late in life.

In the teenage years, failure to spend even $4,000 can easily create a $40,000 full mouth restoration case at age forty or fifty, or embarrassing, health-compromising removal of all teeth and use of dentures at age sixty.

Gum disease is serious business. It worsens the risks of and heightens dangers from diabetes, heart disease, strokes, and dimentia. Ignoring preteen or teen teeth misalignment may virtually guarantee adult medical problems. If there is a genetic history of any of these medical problems we just named, you only worsen the odds of your son or daughter suffering from them by ignoring or postponing needed orthodontic treatment.

Aside from impacting health, a poorly aligned smile can significantly impact your child's comfort. Headaches, toothaches, snoring, drooling, bad breath, and insomnia are all symptoms of a smile that isn't straight, jaws that aren't aligned, or teeth that are too close together or not quite close enough. Oftentimes, however, the mouth is the last place we check for signs of discomfort, loss of sleep, or even a simple headache.

If your child's pediatrician can't figure out why she's not sleeping well or experiencing headaches or even insomnia for which there seems to be no cause, a simple thirty-minute exam at your local orthodontist could provide a clear solution in no time!

Here is what we're told by an awful lot of patients:

"I had wonderful parents, but I sure wish they had found a way to afford the braces I needed and gotten me the care I needed when I was a kid, so I didn't grow up to have this bad smile my whole life and have to deal with all these problems *now*."

Is this how you want your daughter or son talking about you ten, twenty, or thirty years from now? Is this how you want them remembering their childhood? Your parenting?

If that sounds pretty damned pushy, we admit: it is. We kept it in the book for the very simple reason that this is *truly* what we have heard so much over the years, and we are sincere about letting you reflect on it. All parents want to do the right thing. They don't want to let their children down in any way, and we're sure you don't either.

You know, parents just about kill themselves over their kids' college, trying their best to guide the decision, trekking around the country on campus visits, worrying over campus culture, or taking on *serious* debt. Every parent understands what many kids can't— that it's not about the few years of college but rather the forty or fifty years afterward.

We assure you, this is the same. It's not about the bad, humiliating smile and bad bite transformed now, for high school. It's about the many, many years to come. They really can't appreciate that now, but *you* can.

No parent wants their child to suffer, either from teeth that actually hurt, headaches you can't explain, insomnia that affects their daily life, or insecurity your child may be feeling because of a crooked or oversized smile. The fact is, your child's formative years are actually the most sensitive for his or her teeth. Now is the time to pay close attention to your child's smile, behavior, peer relationships, and confidence level.

If any or all are lacking, a qualified orthodontist may help give you and your child the peace of mind you both crave.

The Top Five Reasons People Avoid Seeing the Orthodontist

1. **Patients are afraid it's going to hurt.** Pain is the number-one reason most people avoid going to the orthodontist. However, modern technology—and

choosing the right orthodontist—can ensure that your child enjoys a pain-free orthodontic experience.

2. **Patients are afraid it's going to cost too much.** Not only are most orthodontic procedures more affordable than ever, but insurance, payment plans, and a variety of other financing options make this all but a moot point for most of our patients. Remember, orthodontists aren't in this to get rich, they're here to make sure your child's teeth, smile, and jaw are aligned to make his or her life better—period! We're not going to let something like price get in the way of creating a better, safer, healthier smile for your child.

3. **Patients are afraid it's going to take too long / they're going to miss too much school or work.** Regardless of the type of orthodontic procedure your child needs, time is of the essence. Modern technology and ease of access allows us to work around your child's school schedule with minimal absences. After initial visits, and barring the actual procedure itself, most visits and/or adjustments are routine and can take anywhere from fifteen to forty-five minutes.

4. **Patients do not see the need to take action.** Eroding, crooked, or unaligned smiles can take time to happen, but the time to act is now. Orthodontic irregularities don't just heal on their own or disappear if you ignore them. Your child's smile and overall dental health are too important to ignore out of questions of pain, convenience, or even price.

5. **Patients have been treated in the past with an attitude of indifference.** Let's face it, not all doctors are created equal. Every profession has its "bad apples," and to say dentistry is the exception would be to write fiction instead of fact. There is no room for indifference when it comes to your child's health-care. Find an orthodontic specialist that offers not only state of the art technology for your child, but state of the art service as well. Orthodontic specialists know what it's like to sit in the chair, and should provide every opportunity for patients, especially our younger patients, to feel comfortable, safe, and secure in our care.

Call us at **205-733-2022** or go to **bhamorthodontics.com** to schedule your own Customized Smile Analysis.

Chapter Two

Why Do Kids Need Braces?

ARE BRACES SOMETHING CREATED by orthodontists to make money, like Disney and their extra-charge FastPass? Was it a conspiracy from the very start?

Then and now, there may be some overprescribing and premature prescribing by some doctors. There are bad apples in every orchard. And you know the adage: if all he's got is a hammer, everything (and everybody) looks like a nail.

But there is a very legitimate, clinically documented, and 90 percent of the time, clearly visible reason why some kids, as young as eight, *need* orthodontic treatment and care: malocclusion.

Malocclusion is mostly genetic, so if your daughter or son has it, blame their grandparents. It's a fancy-pants term for all things related to misaligned teeth—teeth growing angled, crooked, and into a too-crowded space. It can be a single tooth, a few teeth, or the whole mouth. As we said, it is mostly hereditary, and your kids didn't get to pick their parents out of a Barbie catalog. There can be other causes too, like early, premature loss of primary teeth, chronic thumb-sucking, or even an accident that seemed to leave no lasting effect at its moment in time.

If your child is suffering from any, several, or all of the following early indicators of malocclusion, consider having them addressed by an orthodontic specialist sooner rather than later:

- **Crossbites**: A crossbite occurs when the jaw deviates to one side with an improper fit of the upper and lower teeth from left to right or front to back. Crossbites can lead to worn and chipped teeth, jaw pain, and asymmetric growth of the jaws. Left untreated, the crossbite will require more extensive treatment later in life and significant jaw surgery in the most-severe cases.

- **Thumb-sucking**: Thumb-sucking habits beginning at the age of seven or older should be corrected immediately in order to prevent severe jaw and tooth alignment problems.

- **Miscellaneous concerns**: There are several associated issues you should also be looking for as soon as your child turns seven in order to intervene early, including the following:

  - permanent teeth that are growing into the wrong spots

  - severely protruded front teeth at risk for injury or causing teasing at school

  - severe crowding with permanent teeth erupting into poor-quality gum tissue

With any of these situations, we can discuss the pros and cons of early intervention and treatment versus waiting until all the permanent teeth are in for braces. If you are anxious about the appearance of your child's teeth or your child is self-conscious about his or her appearance, early treatment might be the best choice. Not only are most orthodontic problems more difficult to correct later, but self-image and personality inhibition can be hard for a person to leave behind. However, if your child is extremely resistant to braces or is not mature enough to be trusted to care for them, delay may be the better choice. In that case, regularly scheduled orthodontic checkups will be necessary.

Having malocclusion does *not* guarantee a child will need braces. Frankly, this is what worries us about nonspecialists like family dentists substituting themselves for orthodontists, and parents letting it happen. They may easily miss an early diagnosis of malocclusion when it could have been treated without braces. Or they may leap to braces as the only way to treat all malocclusion. Either way, you and your child lose.

The first question, then, is: does your daughter or son have or show all the signs they are going to have malocclusion? Second, if so, what—of numerous options—should be done about it? Third, when?

To have all these questions answered early, the first full orthodontic exam should occur early in a child's life. We recommend seven or eight, no later than nine, especially if there is family history of malocclusion. With early and periodic exams by an orthodontic specialist, you may avoid your child's need for braces and/or you may prevent years of suffering and embarrassment related to their teeth and smile.

Waiting will have very serious consequences, often requiring more treatment and higher costs later in life. What most parents fail to realize is that these treatment problems are urgent and should be treated as such. If that ship has sailed, the next best time for a full orthodontic exam is tomorrow at three o'clock.

If your son or daughter does need braces—now or at some predictable future time—the outcome of the exam can lead to *sensible* decisions. If not now, treatment to prevent the need can begin, and also, you can begin saving money for braces or other procedures if necessary later on in your child's life. There is no tooth fairy coming to leave a few thousand dollars underneath his pillow or yours. But if the need must be met three years from now, skipping one Starbucks run a week for those three years can make a hefty dent in the bill to come. Utilizing a Health Savings Account or Flex Spending Account can help, as well. How to fund orthodontic treatment is discussed later in the book.

Let us be emphatically clear. We are *not* in the business of putting braces on any child who doesn't need braces. Our office is *not* a braces store. We're in the business of helping kids and families get the right orthodontic treatment if any is needed, get the right braces if any are needed, and have as perfect a smile and as few oral health problems as possible. We make sure our patients are informed—that's why we wrote this book. In our office, you're never told what to do. You're provided with real information, no medical jargon, plain English, "reasons why," and options. You probably know the term "God complex," referring to a person who acts like he's God—imperious, brusque, and deliberately intimidating to squash questions. You will *not* get that kind of treatment here, from anyone on our team.

Kids do need braces, but not all kids and certainly not the same braces for all. Some kids are better served by other orthodontic treatments instead of or before braces. We will collaborate to figure out what is or isn't needed and what options are best if there is a need for your child.

> Call us at **205-733-2022** or go to **bhamorthodontics.com** to schedule your own Customized Smile Analysis.

Chapter Three

Why Not Just a Dentist?
Why an Orthodontist?

YOU UNDOUBTEDLY ALREADY have a dentist.

Gee, isn't seeing an orthodontist going to cost a lot more?

I'm busy. More appointments?

Do I really need to get orthodontic checkups for my kids?

Don't worry, these are all reasonable questions! It is true that, today, quite a few dentists dance over into our territory, and although they're *not* permitted to claim they're the same as orthodontists or provide orthodontic treatment (beware of any who do), they're able to do things like provide Invisalign and other braces. This can be confusing. Here are the facts.

All orthodontists are dentists and we all graduate from the same dental schools. True enough. But that's where it stops for dentists. Orthodontists go to school for an additional two to three years to become credentialed specialists at diagnosing and providing the best treatment for conditions like:

- difficulties chewing or biting
- constant biting into the cheek, gums, or roof of the mouth
- teeth that meet abnormally or don't meet at all
- teeth grinding or clenching
- crowded, misplaced, or blocked out teeth
- early or late loss of teeth
- teeth grown in badly
- teeth that protrude
- embarrassing personal appearance due to teeth
- facial imbalances
- teeth or jaw misalignment, TMJ
- chronic headaches and migraine
- poor sleep
- speech difficulties (that may never be outgrown or may develop later)

These are *not* dental care issues. They are orthodontic issues.

For *some* things, a generalist or jack-of-all-trades will do. For other things, you know it's smart to seek out the best specialist you can afford. For example, if all your income is in a single W-2 from one employer and you have simple, ordinary deductions, getting your taxes prepared for the cheapest fee at the seasonal H&R Block office that opens up in your neighborhood shopping center is probably fine. But if you have W-2, 1099, and investment income from real estate, depreciation on real estate in several states, own stocks, and you raise iguanas as a money hobby, you're going to get yourself a really good accountant, probably a CPA. If you need the simplest will, leaving everything first to spouse or second to daughter may be okay. But if you are of some means and have several children and maybe also grandchildren as well as charities, you're going to need to see an *estate planning* attorney, not just any attorney—though they all went to the same law schools—but *a specialist in estate planning*.

This is no different.

There are a few things to keep in mind when differentiating between a general dentist and an orthodontic specialist.

First, generalists, or jacks-of-all-trades, tend to work with one-size-fits-all, off-the-rack, standardized solutions. They may be limited to doing only what the computer dictates that they do, without bringing expertise and expert judgment to bear. They're often working with products from only one provider, without being able to select from a full range of options that would work best for you. Specialists, instead, tend to individually and carefully diagnose needs and provide personalized solutions.

Second, generalists and their use of inexpertly applied, standardized solutions tend to be cheaper than the fees of a specialist, but that also places economic pressure on them to do the treatment as quickly and simply as possible, because they've "cut it thin."

In this case, it's worth remembering that the treatment provided has permanent, lifelong, and life-impacting consequences. This concerns your health, future dental or jaw alignment or misalignment issues affecting quality of sleep (which can affect weight, even onset and management of type 2 diabetes and heart disease), as well as self-esteem and social and career success.

> **General Dentist.** A general dentist gives routine checkups, preventive measures, cleans teeth, and fixes cavities. They may not start seeing children until they are seven to ten years old.
>
> **Pediatric Dentist.** A pediatric dentist has two to three years of specialized education beyond dental school. They specialize in providing dental care to children and adolescents, offering checkups, preventive measures, cleanings, and cavities.
>
> **Orthodontist.** An orthodontist has two to three years of specialized education beyond dental school and is an expert at straightening teeth and aligning the jaws. They assess patients and determine the best treatment routes and procedures that need to be taken.

If you can, you want to choose an orthodontist for orthodontic care.

You may ask, *how do I know my doctor is an orthodontist?* It's a good question and a critical one to ask as you seek additional treatment for your child's dental issues.

Only orthodontists can belong to the American Association of Orthodontists (AAO). If you're looking for a local orthodontist, go online and visit **www.braces.org** to find a specialist in your area. This website features not only a searchable database of orthodontists but educational tips, answers and resources to help you on your quest for your child's healthiest smile!

Alternatively, you can ask your doctor if he or she has completed a two- to three-year residency in orthodontics and check with your state dental board to follow up on his reply. Dentists and orthodontists in most states will be registered differently with the dental board.

Do your homework; be a "dental detective" while on the hunt for such vital information. Look for the words "dental specialist in orthodontics," or ask your general dentist for a referral to a specialist. In urban and suburban areas, it will take minimal effort to find a specialist. In more remote, rural locations, your search might take you to another city or town. Don't be afraid to ask your dentist if an orthodontist travels to your town every month to see patients. There's a chance an orthodontist from a larger city comes to your town and works out of another dental office once or twice per month. Looking around can save valuable driving time and money.

One note: there is no disrespect between orthodontists and dentists. As a matter of fact, many orthodontic patients are referred by their dentists. These are great, capable, and caring professionals who know where their expertise begins and ends, and who do not let ego or income opportunity step in front of what they know is best for their patients. Just as the family doctor refers his patients with possible or significant heart disease issues to a cardiologist, and if need be, the cardiologist refers to a surgeon, the best dentists refer patients with orthodontic needs to orthodontists. Orthodontists are required to take two to three years of university education beyond dental school and additional continuing clinical education every year. They must also invest in state-of-the-art technology for their offices (not found in dental offices)—*all for a good reason.*

Even though we orthodontists have the education and training to perform general dentist procedures, we don't. We specialize.

Call us at **205-733-2022** or go to **bhamorthodontics.com** to schedule your own Customized Smile Analysis.

Chapter Four

Choose a Highly Successful Orthodontist

WHY IS THAT IMPORTANT? Wouldn't you get a "better deal" from one barely getting the light bill paid? Maybe. But an overeager orthodontist—or maybe more so, an overeager dentist eager to do braces—might be seeing needs that are more urgent than they really are.

What are some good clues to selecting a great orthodontist?

We've got two: their practice is busy.

We assure you, the ability of advertising to attract orthodontic patients is limited and it's expensive. When you see a really, really busy practice, there are probably a whole lot of patient referrals, and neither kids nor parents enthusiastically refer if they feel they were lied to or treated badly, put in pain, or wound up with results nothing like the digital future-photo they were shown. And they probably wouldn't come to that practice if they had to keep coming back to "fix a few things," or were overcharged. Parents tell parents about great orthodontic practices because we earned their trust and because their kids keep thanking them.

We keep our office very busy. Yes, we advertise. But mostly, these practices thrive by patient referrals. Not that we would anyway, but we don't need to goad you into more and more expensive care than your son's or daughter's situation requires for the best outcome. We don't need to "sell" four more sets of braces this month to win a cruise from the manufacturer—and yes, that stuff goes on in some practices. There's an old cartoon from the *Wall Street Journal* with a bunch of executives in a boardroom at a conference table, one hollering, "Ethics? Ethics? We can't afford ethics!"

This is a business, a business built on ethics and earned trust. And you do *not* just need a doctor to install braces; you need a trust-worthy advisor.

The other clue: a great orthodontist is *not* cheap.

Our fees are calculated to allow for "Cadillac + Care" in every respect, to put no downward financial pressure on how we care for patients and parents, and to *never* cut corners or take shortcuts. We *never* use any material that is "probably good enough."

If we were you, we'd worry if we found an orthodontist that is a lot cheaper anywhere else. If you do find one, know this: behind closed doors they're probably asking, "Can we do this cheaper?" Is *that* the question you want discussed back there, at every step of your child's treatment?

This isn't even like Botox. It's more like cosmetic surgery. There's a science and an art to this. Our staff are all highly trained to produce state-of-the-art outcomes, nothing less. The doctor makes a difference. That's why we tell everybody to get a highly successful orthodontist.

The Top Ten Things You Should Know *Before* Choosing Your Orthodontist

This is something you want to be sure about.

We've just suggested one big consideration: a very successful practice. Here are ten more.

1. Are they a specialist?

Orthodontists are specially trained dentists who take on several extra years of training in order to "straighten teeth," usually by affixing braces to the patient's teeth. You might say we specialize in smiles. Orthodontists also perform dentofacial orthopedics. This is a fancy way to describe how we normalize the structure of a patient's jawbones in order to repair any imbalance in their face. All orthodontists are dentists, but only 6 percent of dentists are orthodontists. Look for the seal of the American Association of Orthodontists (AAO). Only orthodontic specialists can belong to the AAO.

2. Do they treat adults?

Orthodontics is not just for kids! It's important that your orthodontist can treat patients of all ages. Many adults are finding out how a healthy and attractive smile is important to their health and the way they feel about themselves. Others choose to avoid a lifetime of crooked teeth for health concerns or problems with their bite.

3. Do they provide the first visit free of charge?

Most orthodontists offer free examinations for new patients so you and your family can get expert advice about treatment needs, options, and timing before making this important investment. During your first exam and consultation be sure your questions are answered, your concerns are addressed, and you are educated about all of your treatment options. The orthodontist should include digital x-rays during the exam at no charge.

4. Do they offer guarantees? If so, what are they?

No matter which orthodontist you choose, ultimately you are not making a small investment. That being said, wouldn't you want to ensure your orthodontist is going to stand behind their treatment? Of course! We wouldn't have it any other way. In fact, we offer a satisfaction guarantee. If your child has any issues or if you are not satisfied with the treatment, our team of smile specialists will make it right, guaranteed.

5. Are they using the latest technology and treatment options available?

Orthodontics today differs a great deal from years past. Computer-designed braces and wires dramatically increase the precision with which we move teeth and shorten treatment time. Tie-free braces systems have made treatment far more efficient and comfortable. Clear braces offer a cosmetically pleasing alternative, while Invisalign offers patients an entirely brace-free option. Did you know that Invisalign also has a special treatment system just for teens?

Ultimately, you get the best treatment available when you choose us.

6. Does their quoted fee include retainers?

Each orthodontic office has its own fee schedules, and doctors often charge differently for procedures. All orthodontists should offer you a contract that clearly spells out the expenses for your child's treatment before it begins.

Throughout the orthodontic industry, it's common to find out about retainer fees after you start treatment. You should ask your orthodontist about what retainers cost and also if there are any other hidden fees.

7. Do they charge for emergency appointments?

Some minor discomfort may occur with braces. Orthodontists typically provide adjustments for poking wires and loose appliances free of charge. While we do provide these types of adjustments free of charge, you should definitely ask about adjustments and potential costs with your orthodontist before you start treatment.

Keep in mind that if your braces are broken or damaged due to noncompliance with dietary restrictions, this may result in repair charges. If you do your best to avoid breaking your braces and follow the simple dietary guidelines that we will share with you, then you should have no additional costs for adjustments throughout your treatment, even if it's an emergency.

8. Do they make you feel special and comfortable?

Regardless if you are reading this book for your own treatment or for your child's treatment, when you meet with your orthodontist, you should definitely feel comfortable. We strive to make you as comfortable as possible before, during, and after treatment. You are special and we want you to feel special every time you see us.

Particularly important if you are reading this book for the treatment of your child, we also ensure your child feels special every time they visit. Since our doctors are so involved with children and young adults, we can empathize, relate to them, and make them feel comfortable and extra special.

9. Do they have a great reputation?

With the internet, it is extremely easy to pull up ratings and reviews from patients. Simply go to Google and search for orthodontist reviews and ratings in your town.

Additionally, look on the website for video testimonials from actual patients. You can also ask the orthodontist for references.

10. Are they flexible with payment options?

Once you are comfortable and you know specifically which orthodontist you want to treat you or your child, the next question is typically, "How much is this going to cost and how am I going to pay for this?"

We help you understand different payment options from maximizing the most insurance benefits to flex spending accounts to even interest-free payment plans. During the initial exam and complimentary consultation, we will answer all of your questions, including those about our typical cost of braces and the variety of payment options available.

How to Know What Questions to Ask

We've really thought through the questions most parents and patients have—not just the ones they ask, but the ones they don't. This book attempts to cover them all, but again, this is a *personal* matter. The best questions to ask are the ones that matter most to you and your child.

We hope not, but you may be in a position that absolutely requires you to get the minimum essential treatment for the lowest cost. If so, your most important questions are going to be about those kinds of options and about price, and nothing else.

If, however, you are able to make your decision about who you should trust with your child's oral health and smile by many factors, we've included a "What Is Most Important to You?" quiz from Excellence In Orthodontics on the following pages. As you'll see, there are fourteen different items to consider and rank in importance to you. Any can become the questions you ask us and our team or any other orthodontist.

If you have a specific question not answered anywhere in this book, or have a personal and confidential question, you can—with complete assurance of privacy and courtesy—email info@bham-orthodontics.com or call Birmingham Orthodontics directly at 205-733-2022.

There is also a FAQ section at the back of this book.

Of course, a perfect opportunity to get questions answered—yours and your son's or daughter's—is at your exam appointment.

Call us at **205-733-2022** or go to **bhamorthodontics.com** to schedule your own Customized Smile Analysis.

What Is Most Important to You?

Directions: For each **Key Item** below, rank its importance to you from 1 to 5. Then check off whether each type of provider provides that item. When you're done with all 14 Key Items, add up your rankings and review what your final score means about choosing an orthodontist.

	Key Items to Consider in Selecting Your Orthodontist	Rank How Important Each Item Is to You in Selecting Your Orthodontist 1 – Not Important, 5 – Very Important	Check Off If Provided		
			Birmingham Orthodontics	Other Provider	Other Provider
1	Orthodontist and staff committed to expert, thorough diagnosis, and prescription of the best treatment plan customized for my son or daughter	1 2 3 4 5	✓		
2	Avoiding extractions (if possible)	1 2 3 4 5	✓		
3	Avoiding having to wear headgear with braces (if possible)	1 2 3 4 5	✓		
4	Avoiding "metal-mouth" braces (if possible) or utilizing the new type of "invisible" braces	1 2 3 4 5	✓		
5	Having a healthy, pleasing smile that will last a lifetime and protect optimum dental health (not just having straightened teeth)	1 2 3 4 5	✓		
6	Pain-free treatment	1 2 3 4 5	✓		
7	Orthodontist utilizes the most modern, advanced, and proven technology, including computer-aided design and fitting	1 2 3 4 5	✓		
8	Orthodontists and team actively involved in continuing clinical education	1 2 3 4 5	✓		
9	Reducing treatment time to a minimum without compromising results (including total length of treatment term and number of office visits)	1 2 3 4 5	✓		
10	Availability of after-school appointment options	1 2 3 4 5	✓		
11	Treatment coordinator is knowledgeable about insurance coverage and is able to offer flexible payment plans	1 2 3 4 5	✓		

12	Getting the best overall value factoring in thorough diagnosis, customized care, and concern with lifetime health and well-being—not just the cheapest fee	1	2	3	4	5	✔		
13	Smile guarantee	1	2	3	4	5	✔		
14	Orthodontist and team committed to excellence in orthodontics and customer service for both patients and parents	1	2	3	4	5	✔		

Total of Your Rankings

What Your Score Means

50-70   There is no doubt. Birmingham Orthodontics is the right choice for you and your family! It is clear that you place a high value on a comprehensive, "best" approach.

43-49   You are probably also going to be happiest with Birmingham Orthodontics, rather than any other alternative. But this score suggests you aren't completely sure and have some unanswered questions or concerns. Your doctor and the practice's treatment coordinator want no lingering uncertainties on your part, and want to address any and every question. Don't keep anything to yourself. Please ask.

42 or less   Frankly, you may not value the advanced, sophisticated level of clinical care and customer service provided at Birmingham Orthodontics. Cost may be much more important to you than other factors, or very basic service may be all you feel you need. It's perfectly okay. If you choose to shop around, be sure to use this checklist in evaluating other options. Remember, you do want everything right the first time, and you want error-free orthodontics at a minimum.

Chapter Five

What Can I Expect at the Initial Consultation and Exam?

MANY QUESTIONS SURROUND YOUR first visit to a new orthodontist, not the least of which is the subject of this particular chapter: *what will happen at the initial consultation?*

To answer this very common question, and perhaps several others you might not even realize you need answering yet, let us walk you through the typical first office visit, from the initial appointment forward. Your first appointment is scheduled following your initial phone call to your orthodontist's office.

1. **On arrival at the office, you will be greeted by one of our certified treatment coordinators**. She or he is fully prepared to make everything from the first appointment to an entire treatment program go smoothly for you and your child. Your treatment coordinator will manage your relationship with us, from appointment scheduling for your convenience to answering questions.

At the initial visit, your treatment coordinator will review your child's patient information and health history and/or any apparent concerns with you, though this interview and required-by-law paperwork doesn't take long.

2. **Next, your orthodontist will conduct the "Customized Smile Analysis,"** the most complete and thorough orthodontic exam, including teeth, gums, mouth, jaws, and face. Typically, safe digital x-rays are taken of the teeth and surrounding bone and of the jaw structures. Facial photographs, pictures of the teeth and digitalized scans of the teeth may also be made.

The orthodontist will then perform a comprehensive orthodontic examination using the x-rays, photos and digitalized scans, and will present his or her "report of findings." This is a "show-n-tell," in plain English (not medical jargon), of the full state of your child's teeth, gums, mouth and jaws, as well as a diagnosis of any present or anticipated problems that should get orthodontic treatment. If treatment should be needed, your orthodontist will present recommendations and options. This will be an individualized, personalized plan of treatment, not "braces in a box, off the shelf." By this report of findings, you will know:

- what teeth or jaw misalignment or other problems exist or are developing

- what the health and appearance ramifications are of not intervening with treatment

- if braces are needed now or later and which type of braces will be best in your situation

- what the complete treatment program will consist of: things like braces, anticipated length of treatment, and average time of each office visit

- what results will be achieved at the end of treatment

3. **All your questions will be answered**. There are no dumb or embarrassing questions. Every single one of our patients has a question, simple or complex! We do *not* want you or your son or daughter just nodding, then later wondering, "What did he mean by *that?*" or saying, "I wish I'd asked about ..." This is *not* one of those "I'm the doctor—trust me—just do what I say because I said so" offices. Most questions will have been answered by the pre-exam video, other literature provided to you, this book, and your orthodontist's report of findings, but it's a lot to take in. So, any and all questions you have should be asked and answered. Our goal is not just a terrific orthodontic outcome ensuring a healthy, attractive smile, but also your anxiety-free comfort from start to finish.

4. **Finally, your treatment coordinator will explain the costs of the prescribed treatment program and discuss payment arrangements as needed**. In our office, you or your child can get started with treatment with no down payment and low monthly payments. Most of our patients choose to get started with treatment the same day as their initial exam. If no dental work is needed to be done by their general dentist/hygienist, the first of the monthly payments is made and the braces can be placed or an appointment can be made for a more convenient time, whichever is easier. It's that simple! As the saying goes, a journey of a thousand steps begins with the first one, and a task well begun is sooner done!

In total, you should allow about one hour for this entire initial consultation and exam.

If that seems like a lot, keep in mind there are *lifetime* health, appearance, and personality aspects of this. And it's not "installing tires"—not if it's done properly and expertly. Your son or daughter deserves a careful, thorough, and anxieties-eliminated experience. You want to make the best decisions for them.

Frankly, our practice and our process is not for everybody. We attract and "resonate with" parents who are quite serious about their responsibilities and committed to giving their child every possible advantage in life—certainly not unnecessary disadvantages. If you are that parent—and the fact that you took the trouble to obtain and read this book suggests it—then you are going to recognize that this is time well invested in the best possible results.

Call us at **205-733-2022** or go to **bhamorthodontics.com** to schedule your own Customized Smile Analysis.

"Our experience with the orthodontist has been better than we ever expected. My son is so proud of his smile, more and more every day."

—MARY C.

Chapter Six

Shouldn't There Be a Guarantee?

HEALTH CARE IS NOTORIOUS for no guarantees.

Surgeons have a dark-humor insiders' joke: dead patients can't sue.

If you've seen reality TV shows about plastic surgery, like the popular one airing as we wrote this, *Botched*, you know things can go horribly wrong.

Guarantees are controversial in all kinds of health care, including orthodontics. Many doctors are upset by the very idea. One huffed and puffed at us, "What do you think you're doing with this guarantee nonsense? We aren't operating a car shop, installing mufflers and guaranteeing them for five thousand miles. We are doctors, dammit."

His ego was mightily offended. But we doubt you will be, with the challenge of deciding who should be your family's *trusted* orthodontist. So, yes, we think there should be a guarantee! In fact, many guarantees!

1. **If you aren't satisfied with your son or daughter's orthodontic treatment, new smile outcome, or patient/ parent experience,** *our team of specialists will do all we can to make it right, guaranteed.*

2. **Also, the quality of the orthodontic treatment itself is** *guaranteed for life*. If ever the proper teeth alignment originally achieved somehow begins to fail, we will welcome you back and do everything we can to correct the problem.

3. **You also have a safety in numbers guarantee**. The diagnostic and prescriptive methods and state-of-the-art technology and the braces products we use have been used by top orthodontists nationwide to treat over one million patients successfully.

4. **You also have our guarantee that** *every* **orthodontist and orthodontic assistant at our office has been not only academically educated but also** *thoroughly* **trained.** They all follow the same proven method to diagnose needs, plan the best and personalized treatments for every patient, and manage for best results from day one through after-care. All patient care is supervised and reviewed by us. We also invest in frequent state-of-art clinical continuing education for our team exceeding all state licensing requirements. Above and beyond.

5. You also have ***our guarantee of exceptional courtesy and customer service***. Yes, you are our patient, but we can be honest about this—our practice is not just a

health care provider, it is a *business*. As such, it has, in our opinion, one set of responsibilities to you as the parent of a patient and one set to the patient, including telling the whole truth and nothing but the truth, prescribing in the patient's best interest, and delivering the best possible treatment and outcomes. There's also a second, separate set of responsibilities to you as a customer, including access, convenience, responsiveness, and "red carpet service."

These five guarantees are included in your treatment program fee.

For starters, we can guarantee you the best, most thorough orthodontic exam, and we encourage coming in for it now.

Call us at **205-733-2022** or go to **bhamorthodontics.com** to schedule your own Customized Smile Analysis.

Chapter Seven

How to Get More Information

THERE ARE SEVERAL WAYS to get information about an orthodontic practice. First, we want to address the ways we don't recommend.

We don't recommend Yelp. Yelp is, unfortunately, not at all what it seems, and is frequently the subject of lawsuits from business owners, under regulatory scrutiny centered around the poorly policed manipulation of reviews, and has even been accused of the flooding of fake reviews—by "bots" no less! Some companies can use Yelp as competitive warfare while other companies turn around and sell the business owner under negative-review-assault "reputation management services." So, beware! Get the information you need from truly trusted sources.

Google can also be deceptive, though it can be a valuable starting point. Rankings are manipulated by advertisements, websites, YouTube content, and what's called SEO, or search engine optimization. The only thing you know for sure about dentists or orthodontists who come up at the top in Google rankings in your community is that they are good at SEO or, more likely, good at paying somebody who is good at SEO. They're willing to spend money and willing to create a lot of content. Does that equate to certainty of the best diagnostic expertise, treatment, patient care, and customer service? Sometimes. Sometimes not.

So, first, the best thing to do is make certain you get all your questions answered by the orthodontist and the practice's treatment coordinator. Don't hold back. Put them on the spot. Be assertive. Don't feel you have to be deferential to the doctor! Our own goals in this is to have every patient and every patient's parent *fully* knowledgeable about every aspect of the treatment so that they have *zero* anxiety.

Second, visit www.aaoinfo.org. This is the official website of the American Association of Orthodontists, the official, professional organization of educationally qualified orthodontic specialists dedicated to advancing the art and science of orthodontics and dentofacial orthopedics. Their mission is to improve the health of the public by promoting quality orthodontic care and supporting the successful practice of orthodontics. This website can help you decide on the questions you want answers to.

Finally, if you have a quick follow-up visit scheduled, these are wonderful opportunities to either ask questions you may have missed the first time, or to get further details from your orthodontist directly.

Now that we know where to get your most burning orthodontic questions answered, here are some simple tips we've amassed over the years to help you easily and effectively get the information you need:

How to Get Your Questions Answered

Make a list. The easiest way to get what you want is to know it in advance. Make a list of the various questions you have when they arise so you can quickly and easily go down the list to assure you've got the right answers for the right questions.

Bring it with you. Take the list with you when you go for your child's orthodontist visit. This way you have the questions at hand at the right place at the right time. If you're calling in to get answers, you can also have the list ready and tick off one question for every answer you receive.

Double-check. Finally, make sure you have the right answer by double-checking with your orthodontist or his or her treatment coordinator or assistant.

Knowing where to find the information you need is only half the battle; follow these tips and you'll know how to get what you're looking for as well.

Regardless of how many questions you have, or your comfort level with technology, phone calls, or in-person visits, your orthodontist should offer an option that fits your schedule and makes all your unresolved issues crystal clear.

> Call us at **205-733-2022** or go to **bhamorthodontics.com** to schedule your own Customized Smile Analysis.

Chapter Eight

How to Pay For Orthodontic Treatment and Braces

YOU MAY HAVE NEVER needed braces. Or you may have needed them and gotten them. Or you may be among the tens of thousands of people in our generation who needed them but did not get them, perhaps because your family decided they couldn't afford them. Maybe they didn't consider it a priority and probably underestimated the lifelong results of the decision. You may not only have lived with a "hide your smile" habit unnecessarily, but you may have developed chronic jaw pain and headaches, difficulty chewing, or even periodontal disease that could have been prevented.

Regardless of which group you're in—and we hope it's not the third—we hope you will be making the best choices for you, your son or your daughter today, without being hamstrung by the finances. Truth is, parents pay out the same cost for a number of different things not nearly as vital as health or emotional well-being without blinking, mostly because it's paid in installments or just never really *considered*, like the monthly cost for minutes/data on mobile devices, added up for a year or two. The additional insurance cost and other costs when the teenager gets his driver's permit; after all, what's the choice? The cost of braces leaps up and stands there, all at one time. So, it can seem big. And it tempts thoughts of, "maybe later," or, "is this really necessary?"

We hope that in the prior chapters we have succeeded at getting the "is it really necessary?" question erased. If there is visible need or if expert examination by an orthodontist and his explanation of what he finds can show you say it is advisable, it *is* necessary! It won't fix itself. It will probably get worse. It plagues a person's health, emotional well-being, social life, and career. It can link to very serious medical problems. *Necessary* is not really debatable.

Now let's tackle the ugly matter of the money.

We say "ugly" because nobody really likes talking about this. Most orthodontists are nervous about it. Parents are uncomfortable with it. If there is a financial obstacle to treatment, most people are reluctant to admit it, offer other excuses, and then can't be helped by the doctor. We have to trust each other. With us, this discussion is entirely confidential, in a "safe zone." Orthodontists are not Martians, by the way; *we* have kids, college tuitions that loom, and family budgets.

What Is a Reasonable Fee and Cost?

A complete treatment program, including braces, can cost anywhere from $4,000 to $7,500 or so. Most fall in between. As we work very hard to manage the costs for our patients, the cost for full orthodontic treatment at Birmingham is about $4,500. These costs may be variable depending upon the length and complexity of treatment

Adjusted for inflation, these prices are actually *less than* braces decades ago, while the technology and quality has advanced. In costs it can prevent later, it's a bona fide bargain. TMJ treatments are expensive. Cosmetic dentistry work is expensive. Migraine headache drugs are expensive and have side effects.

For this investment, you will be getting the carefully selected, personalized solution to your child's irregularities and problems, prescribed using state-of-the-art digital technology along with the expertise of a specialist, and considerate, compassionate care from start to finish. Your investment includes a varying number of appointments plus the orthodontic appliance itself, after-care, and in our office, certain guarantees.

It's hard to really draw a fair comparison, but if you have any significant net worth, you can easily pay similar fees for the services of an attorney expert in estate planning. Most kitchen remodels cost considerably more. Where real expertise is involved and the stakes of getting it wrong are high, you can't escape professional level fees.

In this case, the $4,000 to $7,500 range is seen as perfectly reasonable by the overwhelming majority of parents that we talk to. Each year, we provide braces of one kind or another to countless patients. Even parents who shook their heads at the cost to start with tell us afterward that having witnessed everything we do to get the absolute best obtainable results, and seeing the outcome itself, they feel undercharged.

While it's never easy to part with such a sum, people do it every day for all sorts of less important things, like their new designer handbag, golf vacation, or suite of living room furniture. They'll pay for it outright or with their favorite credit card (getting the reward points in the bargain). If you put the orthodontic treatment program including braces on a typical credit card at the interest in play as we write this, and you choose to make only the minimum required monthly payment, your monthly payments will be relatively small. Even tight budgets can accommodate this *when it is really important.* It's less than most families pay for their cable and streaming entertainment. For many, if they got all their Starbucks stops consolidated into one monthly bill, it would be more than this!

Birmingham Orthodontics' Interest Free, In-house Payment Plan with No Down Payment and Low Monthly Payments

Since 1993, Birmingham Orthodontics has been providing orthodontic treatment with no down payment and interest free financing. Most orthodontic practices require down payments of 20 to 25 percent or more of the cost of the total orthodontic treatment fee before the braces are placed and then have high monthly fees so the treatment is paid in full before the treatment is completed. This is great for the orthodontist but can be difficult on the patient and their families. Why pay large fees for total treatment and pay large down payments and high monthly payments? These can place a large strain on the family budget and take away some of the joy of receiving a beautiful smile.

We respect families and their budgets. We charge what we feel is a fair fee for orthodontic treatment. We are not trying to be the cheapest orthodontist in town but we are serious about making treatment affordable, providing a great patient experience and giving you a beautiful smile. To qualify for our In-house Payment Plan described above, our patient or their parent/responsible party must:

1. Be employed or show the ability to make the needed payments;

2. Set up monthly auto-draft payments on their credit card or checking account;

3. Be over the age of 21.

The cost of treatment is then spread over the anticipated treatment time to keep the monthly fees low and to allow for treatment to be paid at the time it is completed.

TIP: Most of our patients choose this option. In fact, 60 percent of our patients are so excited about treatment with us that they bring their first monthly payment with them and leave with braces the same day! If this is for you, make sure your teeth are clean and your dentist says they are in good shape and we should be able to get started.

Our patients have found a few other options to be helpful as well (in addition to our In-House Payment Plan).

Health Spending Accounts (HSA) / Flex Spending Accounts (FSA)

The HSA allows you to set aside *pre-tax* dollars to be used for certain medical and health expenses for you or your family. They exist although restricted under the Affordable Care Act (Obamacare) as it stood in July of 2017. By the time you read this, the opportunity may have been expanded, as President Trump suggested. In any case, if you have accumulated money in an HSA, you can probably spend it on orthodontic treatment. If you don't have an HSA, you might want to start one. Information can be found online about existing or new accounts and their rules of use, at www.healthcare.gov.

Other kinds of FSAs are typically set up through your place of employment and similarly enable you to set aside pre-tax dollars for medical expenses. Sometimes, employers match contributions. Again, you can almost certainly tap funds from your FSA for your child's orthodontic care. Check with your employer about this.

If you have a tax accountant, you may want to consult with him about your HSA or FSA.

> **TIP**: How can you make the most out of your employer's flex-pay plan? First, make sure you understand how it works. Second, set aside flex-spending dollars in advance of need, and if possible, make the maximum contributions. Many employers allow higher limits than you'd think without asking, as much as $2,500 to $5,000 per year. Be aware of "family status changes" allowed by your plan that may enable you to change the amount being moved pre-tax from your paychecks to your account anytime during the year rather than just once at the first of the year—so you could bump up the amount in months before the first orthodontic treatment. IMPORTANT: be aware of the balance and the loss of unused funds. In most cases, if you do not use these funds, you lose them, year to year. You usually have three months after the end of the calendar year to submit claims for eligible expenses from the previous year.

Insurance

These days, there are as many different types of insurance plans as there are patients in our office. We can't possibly speak to your unique and personal insurance policy without seeing it first but, in general, our experience tells us that "most" insurance policies cover "some" of your orthodontic expenses.

We realize that answer sounds very vague, but here are a couple of variables you need to answer before an insurance agent can help you determine what, how long, and how many procedures fall under your insurance:

- the type of procedure (braces, Invisalign, etc.)

- the duration of the procedure (two months, six months, a year, etc.)

- the cause of the procedure (a patient presenting with pain, a parent's concern, traumatic injury or accident, congenital birth defect like cleft lip or palate, etc.)

- the nature of the procedure (to correct pain/discomfort, cosmetic, etc.)

We can only partially answer this question, but talking to your insurance agent will help you get the right answers you need.

TIP: Keep an insurance journal of every interaction with your carrier. Write down the date, time of call, name of the person you contacted, and the exact instructions or recommendations following the call. Later, if your insurance company doesn't remember what they told you, you'll have it accurately written down. If they still don't remember, ask them to pull the recorded audio tape from your previous call, so that you can accurately "remind" them of exactly what they told you.

Youth Savings Program

Since many of our patients under ten are not ready to begin treatment, we have a risk-free, pre-payment program called the Youth Savings Program. This provides great saving opportunities such as locking in certain rates or discounts on treatments. The patient or their parent or guardian can determine what monthly amount fits their budget. Thus, when the patient is ready to begin treatment, there will already be a down payment built up, which allows for a lower monthly payment during treatment. The best part is that this is completely risk-free. If the patient moves, decides not to begin treatment, or even gets treatment from a competitor then we offer a complete refund with no questions asked. Even if you are ready for treatment (regardless of age) but you are not able to afford our monthly payments, you can sign up for this risk-free program and make payments until you build up a large enough down payment to allow you to have a monthly payment to fit your budget. Many practices throughout Alabama do not offer such a program yet, but we've found it to be an excellent opportunity for many of our patients.

Loans

If you qualify, we offer iCare Financial, which can provide an unsecured, signature-only loan for the treatment program, with repayment over twelve to sixty months. You don't need to go anywhere else to apply or do paperwork; we can take care of it in our office.

If you have equity in your home, the lowest-cost loan option may be a home equity line of credit or second mortgage. See your own bank, or check out RocketMortgage at rocket.quickenloans. com. As of this writing, mortgage interest is at record lows.

Obviously, a private loan from a family member can be the easiest option. A lot of preteens' and teens' important orthodontic care is financed at the Bank of Grandma and Grandpa.

What If You Really, Really Can't Afford Braces?

We have compiled a list of eighteen ways you may be able to substantially reduce the cost of braces. Frankly, some of them are less than ideal, and most are not available through our office, but they could be helpful if your back is really up against a financial wall.

1. **Get braces in April or November and see if you can save a little extra by paying in full.** These are the months that orthodontists are the least busy, and it's when we have our most meetings (April–May). In November, everyone is getting ready for the holidays or the office is closed the week of Thanksgiving. By scheduling during the "off season," you can often find better deals with willing orthodontists.

2. **See if you can get a discount for not breaking any brackets.** Believe it or not, most orthodontists would happily take $100 off your final bill if you don't break any appliances throughout treatment!

3. **New technology; better pricing.** See if you can be one of your orthodontist's first patients with a new technology and save some money on the lab fee or receive a discount for being a teaching case.

4. **See if your local dental school has an orthodontic program.** The treatment at such institutions is supervised by orthodontists (most of whom practice in the surrounding area). While you might spend a lot more time in the chair as a teaching case, if you have the time, it might be well worth the wait because you can save up to *half the cost of traditional braces.*

5. **Ask your insurance plans when they send out their fee schedules to participating providers.** If the insurance company updates their fees or the orthodontist raises his or her fees to keep up with the cost of inflation, it might be around November in preparation for the next year.

6. **See your dentist every four to six months.** While you're wearing your braces, the extra cleaning each year can prevent tooth decay, a costly item to repair.

7. **Get your flex spending dollars in order with your employer.** If you set money aside in a flex plan, it may be "tax-free," but it comes with some stipulations: namely, you have to use it before the end of the year or else you lose it.

8. **See if you can get a second set of retainers from your orthodontist at the end of treatment.** Sometimes getting two sets of retainers at the same time can be cheaper than buying a second set later in life when you lose or break your first set.

9.   **See if your husband or wife has an insurance plan that covers braces.** Be sure to enroll in the plan with enough time to spare before your child needs braces, so that the procedure is not denied by your insurance company due to a waiting period.

10.   **Ask for flexible financing options.** When you boil it down to the basics, your orthodontist really just wants to help you. Regardless of his specialty, your doctor spent way too much time in school *not* to love what he does. If you're easy to work with, keep your teeth clean, and avoid breaking your braces while you're wearing them, he or she will probably be thrilled to help you finance the care, or find another way to afford the investment.

11.   **Do you have multiple kids in treatment?** If so, take advantage of that fact and see if you can get a family discount.

12.   **If finances are extremely tight, you should check out the organizations that orthodontists have created to help provide pro-bono care, such as Smiles Change Lives.** There are even more foundations like this if you have a cleft palate or other facial anomalies, like the Rheam Foundation for Cleft and Craniofacial Research.

13.   **School auctions, churches, or public service entities will often receive donations from local orthodontists wishing to donate a case to the school or organization for a fundraiser.** Checking around local school newsletters or church bulletins for their upcoming silent auctions could be a great find! If you're unwilling to leave such things to chance, call your local schools or churches and

ask them specifically if they have such a fund and, if so, how to apply/qualify.

14. **If you're thinking about a career change, apply at your local orthodontist's office.** Most orthodontists offer free braces to their staff and their children as an employee benefit! (And you never know, you could love your career *and* your child's new braces!)

15. **Military personnel, schoolteachers, and firefighters sometimes receive special courtesies in dental and orthodontic offices throughout the year.** Keep your ears open and you might save a few bucks or at least get a donation from the orthodontist to your organization.

16. **This tactic won't save you any money, but it could earn your organization or business some money if you have a newsletter, sports team, fund-raiser, or special event that needs a sponsor.** Ask your orthodontist. Most orthodontic offices are huge supporters of the communities in which they practice and would probably love to advertise with your organization.

17. **Got taxes?** Good! Why not use your tax refund to help pay for treatment in full and ask for a courtesy on the average fees associated with financing a full orthodontic case? In some areas, you can save as much as 10 percent on the cost of braces by simply saving your pennies and paying the entire bill at once, up front.

18. **Ask for more flexible financing through a third-party credit company like Chase Healthcare Advance, through CareCredit, or by using in-house financing through your**

orthodontist. Most orthodontists will accept a reasonable down payment and split the remaining amount into easy monthly payments for your convenience. With automated withdrawals from a checking or savings account, you might be able to stretch the monthly payments out over a longer period to make each payment lower. Just don't be shocked if your orthodontist asks you to approve a credit check. A little homework up front can be well worth the effort when your monthly orthodontic bill is lower than your cell phone bill!

There's no doubt about it; braces can be expensive. However, now that you're armed with these eighteen massive, budget-saving tips, you won't need to decide between braces and your budget ever again!

Call us at **205-733-2022** or go to **bhamorthodontics.com** to schedule your own Customized Smile Analysis.

Chapter Nine

What Are the Treatment Options?

IF YOUR CHILD IS ready for orthodontic care, one of the first discussions to have with your orthodontist is which procedure is right for him or her; there might be more options than you had ever imagined.

If you're like most people, you associate orthodontists with braces, but these days, that is just one arm of what an orthodontist does. Here are some of the services most orthodontists will provide their patients with during the course of routine treatment:

- metal, tie-free braces

- lingual braces placed behind your teeth

- Invisalign clear removable aligners

- clear braces

- expanders to match jaw size and tooth size

- habit appliances to eliminate thumb sucking

- space maintainers

- retainers to prevent crowding and shifting of teeth

- headgear to help correct jaw alignment

- functional appliances to help improve facial balance

- early treatment and growth modification

- customized appliances designed uniquely for each patient

- surgical orthodontics to correct or improve facial imbalances

While many of these services may seem self-explanatory to you, several will probably not. In the following pages, we will try to elaborate on several of them, including:

- crossbite correction

- metal braces

- clear braces

- Invisalign

Crossbite Correction

As your child's teeth begin to grow in, there's a *lot* more at work than mere gum lines, tooth fairies, and molar size. How the jaw is shaped, when it develops, and even how "normally" it develops can all affect the placement and comfort of your child's teeth.

When the upper and lower teeth grow at different rates, or even when the lower jaw grows disproportionately with the upper jaw, something known as a "crossbite" can occur.

Your child might have a crossbite if, for instance, the lower jaw is out of line with the upper jaw (kind of like a box that won't close right because one of the hinges is bent).

Or perhaps on the right side of your child's mouth, the lower teeth "stick out" a little farther than the top teeth, making the upper teeth on that side overlap in turn.

Or maybe your child's upper and lower jaws are out of alignment so instead of the top and bottom front teeth meeting "naturally" as they should, the front teeth fall somewhat behind the lower teeth. This would be the reverse of an overbite.

As you might imagine, any or all of these developments can lead to short- and long-term discomfort for your child.

How, When, and Why Crossbites Form

You might be amazed to find out how many ways a crossbite can form as your child grows and develops during his or her formative years. Heredity is one key to jaw growth, or alignment, as is the size of your child's developing jaw.

Another factor that can contribute to the development of a potential crossbite is if it takes your child too long to lose his or her baby teeth. In some extreme cases, in fact, if it takes too long for your child to lose his baby teeth, another set of teeth can grow in behind them, throwing the alignment off and contributing to a crossbite.

Believe it or not, something as basic as whether your child breathes through her nose or her mouth can also contribute to a crossbite. While most children breathe through their noses, some children develop a habit early on of breathing through their mouths instead.

In children who breathe through their noses while they're sleeping, the tongue naturally rests on the roof of the mouth, promoting natural and proper upper jaw growth. When young children breathe through their mouths, however, the tongue relocates from the roof of the mouth to the bottom, removing that extra support and potentially contributing to reduced upper jaw bone growth; this can create the crossbite we spoke of previously.

How Can I Spot a Crossbite?

Although it sounds severe, and even painful from the description provided earlier, the effects of a crossbite can take time to manifest themselves. Still, here are some of the telltale signs your child might be cultivating, or already suffering from, a crossbite:

- snoring

- difficulty breathing

- chewing on one side of the mouth or the other

- signs of an underbite

- if your child's chin seems "off center" or disproportionate

How, When, and Why to Correct a Crossbite

Where should you start looking for treatment if you're concerned about your child's jaw development after reading this section? If you suspect your child might have a crossbite, approach your family dentist about a recommendation for a specialist such as an orthodontist.

There are many possible treatments available for a crossbite, and your orthodontist can work with you closely to make the right and specific decisions for you and your child.

When should you start? We believe you know our standard answer when it comes to questions like this one: *as early as possible*! The same way an auto mechanic would tell you to take care of that oil leak, bulging tire, or faulty timing belt—sooner rather than later. We and our colleagues in orthodontics will always favor early treatment to later.

Crossbites are often closely linked with other orthodontic issues, such as teeth alignment, jaw size, and growth, so naturally, the sooner you address any or all of these issues, the better.

Finally, why should you address a crossbite? Crossbites can lead to pain, discomfort, and a lack of confidence as your child begins to feel insecure or even ostracized because of this very treatable, very normal series of jaw and teeth developments.

Not only can crossbites become physically uncomfortable if left untreated, but if the misalignment or root cause of the bite isn't fixed early in childhood, then the child's appearance and, ultimately, confidence could be affected as the crossbite becomes more pronounced in adolescence.

Metal Braces

The fact is, metal braces still have a valued place in the orthodontic world, and despite advances and breakthroughs of products like Invisalign and even clear braces, they aren't going extinct anytime soon! This is because metal braces are very strong and can withstand most types of treatment. Today's metal braces are smaller, sleeker, and more polished than ever before.

"Our son has a lot of anxiety about visiting any doctor, but the transition into the orthodontics world was very easy and painless for our family. Thank you for all that you do to bring beautiful smiles to our family and many, many more!"

—MOLLY H.

Older, traditional metal braces require an elastic o-shaped rubber band, called a ligature, to hold the arch wire onto the bracket. These elastic ties collect more plaque and bacteria, making it harder for patients to clean the teeth and gums.

You may have heard of "speed braces." These are sometimes also referred to as "self-ligating brackets" or "tie-free braces." Self-ligating means that the brackets do not need the little o-shaped rubber bands (ligatures) or metal tie wires to hold the arch wire onto the bracket. Several companies have developed braces for holding the wires in place without ligatures.

By using self-ligation technology, the brackets allow the wire to slide back and forth. This advancement allows for fewer adjustments and fewer appointments. These types of braces do not need rubber bands to hold the arch wire in place, although most patients still prefer to have colored o-ring ties on their braces. They use a "door" to secure the arch wire to the bracket. They're smaller than traditional metal and less food gets trapped around them when you eat.

Your orthodontist might use an advanced self-ligating bracket that does not require physical tightening of the wire to the braces. It's a twin bracket made of metal or clear ceramic and utilizes a special built-in clip. The pressure from specific types of arch wires activates the clip and delivers specific amounts of force to each tooth, resulting in fast, directed results.

Naturally, orthodontists are very excited about the hygiene benefits of these self-closing or tie-free metal braces. Patients are excited that their braces are small, smooth, and friction-free, and will straighten their teeth in fewer visits with less discomfort than braces with wires that are "tied-in."

Clear Braces

Ceramic braces are very strong and generally do not stain. Two popular brands are Clarity, made by 3M Unitek, and Radiance, made by American Orthodontics. Adults like to choose ceramic because they "blend in" with the teeth and are less noticeable than metal. These are the type of braces actor Tom Cruise had.

Today's clear braces can be very aesthetic as they no longer stain as easily with certain foods and drinks.

Adult Orthodontics

It's not uncommon for individuals who have undergone orthodontic treatment earlier in life to find their teeth have drifted out of alignment over the years. Most adults won't think twice about bleaching their teeth to roll back the effects of time. Yet few think about the role orthodontics can play.

Adults of all ages can enjoy the same cosmetic and health benefits of properly aligned teeth with appliances like clear braces or clear aligners such as Invisalign.

Improperly aligned teeth can do more than undermine your confidence. They can make proper cleaning and brushing more difficult, contribute to enamel loss, and even set the stage for more significant problems down the road. Fortunately, discrete treatment with clear braces can help keep you aligned with a healthy, happy lifestyle.

The Solution Is Clear

Orthodontists believe every individual has the right to live their life with a smile they truly love, particularly children. Healthy, straight, and attractive smiles make your child happier and more self-confident. And isn't that what we all want for them?

Orthodontic treatment with clear, self-ligating braces can help you achieve the smile of your dreams faster, easier, and more discretely than you ever imagined. Embrace the confidence that comes with beautifully aligned teeth and put your smile on display. Schedule a consultation and ask if these braces are right for you.

Invisalign

Invisalign is a widely advertised, well-known, and popular orthodontic product. Kids and adults often know about it and ask parents and doctors for it by name. For many, it's as good an option as any other and sometimes even the best option.

Invisalign uses advanced, proprietary 3-D computer-imaging technology to "map" the entire span of treatment, from the present teeth alignment to the desired positioning, alignment, and smile. Clear aligners are custom made and based on the 3-D imaging. Invisalign has many features that have helped make it such a popular choice. The aligners are removable, even before a snack or meal as well as for general hygiene. There are no metal brackets or wires. Office visits for adjustments throughout the treatment program are fast, easy and painless. The thermoplastic aligners are virtually invisible. Over four million patients have been treated with Invisalign, and there is even a special Invisalign system for teens.

If you would like a patient info kit just about Invisalign, we'll be happy to send it to you. Email your request to info@bhamorthodontics.com or call 205-733-2022.

Because Invisalign is computer mapped, there's sometimes the idea that anybody can install Invisalign and that all practitioners using Invisalign are the same. We have an important warning about this: during each stage of the complete treatment, only certain teeth are allowed to move. Which teeth move in what order, and the amount of time (days/weeks) needed for each successive set of aligners differs for each patient. *This* is what you rely on an expert orthodontist specializing in youth and adult care to decide. At the start, we determine whether you, your son or your daughter are good candidates for the Invisalign approach, or if they would be better served with different braces. You have to rely on *somebody* to tell you. We promise you, there are people who've been hurried to Invisalign who were not good candidates for it.

Invisalign Teen

Much like the standard adult version, the Invisalign Teen System lets you do it the modern, hygienic way. Your new smile is created with the most innovative technology—a series of clear aligners that are custom-fit to your teeth.

The first thing you should know is that an average treatment takes about one to two years. Plus, your treatment can begin even if you don't have all of your permanent teeth. Invisalign Teen was designed to meet your needs.

Invisalign Teen aligners will snap on your child's teeth easily. They are comfortable and practically invisible. Invisalign Teen allows for permanent teeth to grow gently while continuously moving teeth in small increments. Aligners are worn for about two weeks and then swapped for a new pair.

Invisalign Teen aligners have a "Blue Dot Wear Indicator," designed to show an estimation of wear time. The dot is designed to fade until it's clear over a two-week period if you wear your aligners properly (meaning for twenty to twenty-two hours every day).

Invisalign Teen is designed to custom-fit to your child's teeth and go with his or her lifestyle. During your treatment, your child can keep smiling, playing sports, eating what he or she wants, and brushing and flossing normally because the aligners are removable. Plus, unlike traditional braces, the aligners are made of smooth plastic and move teeth gradually.

The aligners are replaceable if lost. That's right; you get up to six free individual aligners.

After your child's Invisalign Teen treatment, you may find his or her self-confidence boosted by their new smile and the change in their appearance. Some people even feel that way during the treatment. As you know, smiling has many benefits. It can help your child make a strong impression in lots of different social situations—at school, at work, or at a party.

Invisalign Teen really works. It helps correct a broad range of dental and orthodontic issues. You can get a confident smile without metal bands, brackets, or wires. It works on many kinds of conditions, including overly crowded or widely spaced teeth, crossbites, overbites, and underbites.

We've used Invisalign to successfully transform the smiles of many patients, but we do not prescribe it to everybody. After all, *popularity* should not govern medical care!

Trustworthy, Objective Advice

Our office is *not* "in the pocket of" or obligated to any of these providers of different braces products and technologies. We select and recommend what we believe is *the* most appropriate and beneficial choice for your child. We are happy to discuss the pros and cons of different ones, if your child has heart set on, say, Invisalign, because that's what a friend has, or based on information you've obtained.

Candidly, these manufacturers vary in price to the orthodontist (or dentist) based on volume purchase benchmarks, incentivizing concentration of as much use as possible to one product. Awards are given out to the highest volume buyers and users. It's borderline unseemly. It introduces temptation into the diagnostic and prescriptive process, and we'll never let the practice bow to such incentives and temptations. The number-one rule here is: what is absolutely best for the patient?

Call us at **205-733-2022** or go to **bhamorthodontics.com** to schedule your own Customized Smile Analysis.

Chapter Ten

How Difficult Is Living with Braces

REMEMBER, THIS ISN'T 1982. Or 1992. Today's braces aren't anything like yours if you had them decades ago. Today's orthodontic care is far more advanced, more sophisticated, and more patient-centered than any prior generation has experienced. If you had traditional metal braces twenty years or so ago, you experienced medieval torture. The dungeon is gone too, replaced by ultra-modern, comfortable, and patient-friendly offices. Out of the dark, into the light!

Living with braces is *not* going to be anywhere near as difficult as you might imagine.

Let's look at a few specific concerns.

Brushing and Hygiene

Modern braces, whether they're metal, flexible, or "invisible," are all actually made to fit the individual and facilitate easy, painless, thorough brushing. This means your child brushes pretty much the same as he would if he didn't have braces.

Here are some simple tips you can share with your child for the best results when brushing with braces on:

- Brush your teeth with a soft or medium nylon toothbrush after you eat and before bed.

- Brush, rinse, and look; if you find any areas that are not clean, brush them again.

- Brush your gums as you brush your teeth (massage and stimulate).

- Take extra care in the area between the gums and the braces because food caught and left there can cause swollen gums, cavities, discomfort, and permanent teeth stains.

- If no toothpaste is available, brush without.

- If you are unable to brush, rinse your mouth vigorously with water.

- Replace your old toothbrush when it gets worn out.

- It's absolutely essential you continue regular visits to your family dentist for checkups and cleanings throughout your orthodontic treatment!

Depending on the age of your child, you, the parent, may need to supervise the first few brushings with the braces in place. You should *not* have a whining, resistant, difficult child on your hands because of any of this. It should be painless, simple, and routine.

Forbidden Foods Your Child Must Avoid

After your child's orthodontic appliance/braces have been placed, the teeth are usually "tender" and sensitive for as few as three to as many as ten days: a *short* time. During these few days, softer foods are recommended: soups, macaroni, spaghetti, eggs, fish, Jell-O, yogurt. As needed, Tylenol or Advil are adequate in relieving any discomfort, taken an hour or so before eating.[3] Warm saltwater rinses can be helpful. We also provide a "soft white wax," a safe topical that eases gum discomfort.

For the entire duration of the braces being in place, we'd advise you to stay away from hard and sticky foods that can damage braces and may lengthen the time they have to be worn or even require extra office visits. Sugar-rich foods can make hygiene harder and cause calculus build-up and cavities. You're probably already monitoring and limiting your child's intake of such foods, so there's really nothing new under the sun here. But, for the record, here are the "featured items" that should be avoided during orthodontic treatment and wearing of braces:

1. **Rock-hard foods**: ice (don't chew ice!), nuts, popcorn (has hard kernels inside), peanut brittle, rock candy, whole

---

3   Prescription pain pills with dangerous side effects are not needed. Any ortho-
    dontist or dentist easily prescribing such drugs is not to be trusted. As you are no
    doubt aware from the news, opioid addiction is rampant. Pain drugs are, contrary
    to early assertions by their manufacturers, proving to be extremely addictive for
    many people after nominal and legitimate use. We can't emphasize enough—we
    practice truly pain-free orthodontics.

apples and carrots (unless cut into bite sized pieces), corn on the cob, hard pretzels, hard rolls, hard taco shells.

2. **Extra-sticky foods**: Jolly Ranchers or Starbursts or similar candies, bubble gum, taffy, and sticky Cinnabon rolls.

3. **Very chewy foods**: pizza crust, beef jerky, gummy bears. Note: no chewing on pencils or pens.

4. **Super sugary foods and drinks**: soda pop with sugar, ice cream, most cookies, and cake. Yes, this is the worst of the forbidden foods. Some kids will give you a tough time. But there are sugar-free versions of all these kinds of foods, to be made, baked, or store-bought.

We will speak about this with your son or daughter and give them a printed list, but *you* will have to reinforce, monitor, and provide some substitute foods to prevent mutiny or months of sulking. Most kids get it, though. When they understand how short or long the number of weeks of wearing braces will turn out to be, how comfortable or uncomfortable wearing them is, how maintaining hygiene while wearing them is, and how their results are linked to them staying away from the short list of harmful foods, they are pretty responsible about it. Most parents who are initially really worried about this tell us later it wasn't the horror show they'd imagined.

Emergencies, Injuries, Travel, and Time Away from Home

Many "emergencies" actually aren't and can be easily and safely remedied at home. We will go over proper care of your braces when they are placed and you can always access the same information at our web site, 24/7, 365 days/year.

Common emergencies include the breaking of some part of the braces, eating something particularly damaging—even a McDonalds bun full of sesame seeds might feel like an emergency, or, early, a feeling of discomfort that worries something serious might be wrong. These are the sort of things addressed in the "What to Do" instructions.

If you do run up against an emergency that isn't easily managed with these instructions or if you can't wait for regular office hours, we have a special phone number to call that routes to a knowledgeable staff member directly.

If your family or son or daughter are away from home and, say, they chomp down on a piece of toffee and break a piece of their braces, there is *always* a remedy. You are *not* going to cut your vacation short and rush to the airport! Again, often a remedy provided by our instructions can meet the urgent need until everybody gets back home. With some types of braces, we can FedEx temporary replacements. We also belong to a network of orthodontists with offices throughout the United States, which we can utilize in *the extremely rare instance* when getting to an orthodontist immediately is vital.

Here is just how good the appliances themselves and our management of orthodontic treatment has gotten. In 2016 to 2017:

- Ninety-eight percent of patients required *no* extra office visits for repairs, adjustments, care, or emergencies beyond their regularly scheduled office visits per their treatment plan.

- Eighty-five percent of patients called with questions, worries, or emergencies that were handled simply by advice and home remedy and/or waited without harm until the next regularly scheduled visit.

- Only 2 percent of patients had some problem or emergency requiring an extra, unscheduled office visit or express delivery of a temporary "patch" or solution to braces broken by sports, play, or other injury.

Sports

Speaking of injuries, the question of sports versus braces worries kids and parents alike. These days, kids are *very* active in organized and school sports, some starting one as another's season is ending. You know this; you are coordinating the schedules and working as their unpaid chauffeur.

Good news: for every sport and every level of play, there is either an inexpensive off-the-shelf mouth guard or a slightly costlier, custom-fit mouth guard to provide an extra, suitable level of dental protection and to protect the braces themselves. In some sports, additional face masks or other equipment normally treated as an option can be added and used during the time period of the orthodontic treatment. Ask us for guidance for your child and their sport(s). Some mouth guards even come with insurance against dental injury, covering financial costs.

We have thought this through! For example, research reported in *Clinics in Sports Medicine*—from the Department of Neurology at Boston University School of Medicine—examined uses of different kinds of mouth guards and the rate of sports-related concussions. There was no significant difference in concussion risks found tied to different types of mouth guards. We can select the best one for your child, their sport, and the level of play.

This, by the way, is typical of a good orthodontic specialist: attention to *every* detail. They should have a good knowledge of every ramification of wearing braces, clinical and technological advancements, and every patient or parent need. To be blunt, it's a practical impossibility for a general dentist to give the braces work he does on the side anywhere near this same level of all-in focus.

By the way, there are collegiate and pro athletes—even NFL players—getting orthodontic treatment and even wearing braces. If they can, your child can! You do *not* need the drama of stopping your child from playing the sports they're committed to because of their orthodontic treatment.

See, this *isn't* going to be difficult!

Tips for Helping Your Child Adjust to a Life with Braces

- **All the cool kids are doing it (or soon will be):** Braces are a very popular appliance during the middle school and high school years. Rather than focus on how he or she feels wearing braces, encourage your child to begin actively looking for other kids who are wearing braces. Chances are, they'll find lots more than they ever imagined!

- **Even famous people do it:** Gwen Stefani. Prince Harry. Drew Barrymore. Tom Cruise. Dakota Fanning. Danny Glover. Brett Favre. Terrell Owens. The list of famous people who've worn braces—many of them as adults—could fill half this book. Share with your child how even the most famous people in the spotlight sometimes need a little help through braces.

- **Fast forward:** Many orthodontists provide a "before and after" consultant's session, much like a plastic surgeon. Digital pictures are often used to portray what the child's teeth might look like once the braces have been removed. Have your child focus on the "after" when he or she gets down about the "before" shots!

- **Be prepared:** Finally, create a "master list" of things your child likes to do, things that make them feel special, confident, brave, calm, relaxed, or excited. If you notice them feeling down, consult your list and make plans to do something special in the near future to boost their confidence level back to where you know it belongs!

Call us at **205-733-2022** or go to **bhamorthodontics.com** to schedule your own Customized Smile Analysis.

Chapter Eleven

Life After Braces: Retainers

SO, YOUR CHILD'S BRACES are off and they're ready to live a life full of confidence and good oral health. They may think, *I'm free! I'm free!* Well, not quite yet.

The selection of the right braces, the expert orthodontist, and the compliant wearing of the braces gets us about three-fourths of the way to where we want to be: a well-aligned, as-perfect-as-possible, healthy smile for life.

But after braces, there are retainers.

While many patients are understandably eager to be done with braces once they come off, the fact is, retainers do as much work—if not more—than the braces themselves. Straight teeth in proper alignment have to stay that way, and for that, retainers are a big help.

When the braces are removed, teeth can still shift if not helped through a period of adjustment to settle in. Retainers gently but purposefully remind the teeth to stay straight during this adjustment period. It's advised that nearly all patients who've gone through the time, work, and expense of braces will want to use fixed or removable retainers for months or years or even for life and continue to schedule regular orthodontic checkups. Some dentists doing braces won't tell you this, but we will. Years ago, clinicians believed that once teeth were straightened by braces, they would simply stay that way forever. New science says otherwise. In fact, teeth position shifting as we age is to be expected. Teeth naturally shift to the middle and crowd. So, retainers are actually extremely important in maintaining the new smile from braces. Any claims otherwise, by some "brand" of braces or any doctor, are flat-out false.

Retainers can play a role in:

- closing any gaps that may remain in the bite

- correcting any speech problems—sometimes occurring with a new bite or jaw position

- tongue thrust—where the tongue slips under the teeth while talking

- bruxism—grinding teeth while sleeping

As you can see, there's a lot more to this than just "installing and removing braces."

In post-braces monitoring and checkups, we tend to decide on the best kind of retainer for your child before the removal of the braces. Growth of the jaw following treatment (yes, the jaw is still growing in adolescents, to age eighteen or so), stabilization of the gums and bone tissues, pressures from lips and tongue, and other factors tell us what type of retainer should be worn and for how long. Retainers are made out of rubber, plastic, and sometimes, still, metal. They are custom made and fit as part of the complete orthodontic treatment. However, after the initial orthodontic exam, at the same time the best braces are being selected, it's usually possible, with a good degree of certainty, to predict the type of retainer(s) your child is going to need, and we're happy to share that information with you at that time.

Some retainers are invisible or nearly invisible. There are clear plastic retainers. A *fixed* retainer is typically placed on the inside/back surfaces of the lower front teeth. A fixed retainer may be used until lower jaw growth is complete and then no longer needed. When your child hears "retainer" he will most likely picture a *removable* retainer. These make hygiene easy, are easily removed and cleaned daily, and can be removed for a sports activity. There are even "fashion retainers" now—popular with kids of different ages—in school colors, and some even with pictures on them!

This is an important part of braces aftercare and part of the complete orthodontic treatment program personalized for your child.

Call us at **205-733-2022** or go to **bhamorthodontics.com** to schedule your own Customized Smile Analysis.

Chapter Twelve

Let's Celebrate!

HAVING TO WEAR BRACES can last for six months to two years or more in certain cases. During the time your child has them, they may have moved from child to preteen or preteen to teen, at times feeling embarrassed by having them, and possibly missing out on some things. They probably gave up favorite foods and snacks. They at least had to be super-conscious of what they ate and didn't eat. It's been a long time since they could sink their teeth into an apple!

You endured whatever complaining there was. You traded time to the office visits. You dealt with the "uh-oh!" and the "now what did you do?" emergencies if there were any. And, of course, you paid the bill.

We like to see our patients celebrate getting their braces off. There are so many ways your child can celebrate, everything from writing a journal about their experience to recording a video that shares their experience and shows their new look.

Here are a few options your child may want to consider:

- **Throw a party**. Throwing a "braces are off" party is a great way to celebrate. They can invite their friends over, put out the foods that they've been longing for, and they can enjoy showing off those new straight teeth. Their friends will love being able to take part in the celebration.

- **Plan a photo shoot**. Your child deserves to show the world their new beautiful smile! Plan a photo shoot, so they can be one-on-one with a photographer and put their best smile forward. They'll get some great shots and can show all their friends on social media their new look.

- **Chew some gum**. Your child might have wanted to have gum for the longest time. Although it's not the best habit, they can take an afternoon to chew some gum and feel guilt and worry free. Chew to your heart's content!

- **Go caramel**. Now is the time your child can sink their teeth into something like a caramel apple. No more avoiding the caramel and cutting the apple into bite-sized pieces. Nope, they can actually eat a full caramel apple, right off the stick! They can get one at the mall or a carnival or even make one themselves. Either way, they'll love being able to bite into that sticky gooey sweetness worry free!

- **Picnic in the park**. Weather permitting, a picnic in the park will make for a fun celebration. Take some of your child's favorite outdoor games, invite the friends, and have a cooler filled with icy drinks. On the grill, you can plan for things like corn on the cob that your child had to largely avoid while wearing their braces. It will make for a memorable afternoon!

- **Have a potluck dinner**. Have your child's friends and family each bring a dish people with braces have to take precaution with. This will give them the chance to learn a little more about what you went through, and it'll be fun to see what options they come up with. Ask each of the guests to write down a comment about your child with or without her braces. Your potluck will be filled with interesting dishes, laughs, and a good time!

- **Relax**. What could be better than spending a couple of hours being pampered, or perhaps a round of golf or fishing out on the lake? Not much! Take your child out—celebrate them making it through their treatment. They'll walk out feeling and looking great!

Doing some of these things, such as chewing gum, may still not be good for your child's teeth or their body overall. But doing it on a special occasion, and not making a habit out of it, won't cause any harm.

Of course, nobody can celebrate unless we *started*. There really is no time like the present.

Call us at **205-733-2022** or go to **bhamorthodontics.com** to schedule your own Customized Smile Analysis.

Chapter Thirteen

What About My Smile?

MOM, DAD, WE'RE NOT going to kid you: if braces and/or orthodontic treatment was advised when you were eight or ten or twelve and, for whatever reason, it didn't happen, and you now have misaligned teeth, periodontal problems because of them, a smile you often hide, and/or jaw/TMJ pain, it may *not* be an easy fix. It may *not* even be fixable with orthodontics or braces. But, often to the surprise of adults, braces—including invisible braces—can do a significant amount of good for people thirty, forty, or even fifty years old. You may still be able to go from an embarrassing smile you often hide to a beautiful smile you love! You'll also be able to enjoy better oral health, gently and gradually, over six to twelve months without having teeth pulled and without surgery. Many adults see ten years of age disappear from their faces!

The only way to know what the options are is with a complete, expert orthodontic exam.

While some offices may not actively seek adult patients, many will treat a lot of parents of patients, just like you, and a number of them come from referrals. You can arrange for your exam by speaking to any of the treatment coordinators at the office.

It's important to get your son or daughter the orthodontic care they need at the earliest time they are known to need it and for it to be the best care available. When that doesn't happen, it often comes around to really bite that person later in life!

Please don't ask them to hide their smile!

Call us at **205-733-2022** or go to **bhamorthodontics.com** to schedule your own Customized Smile Analysis.

"After years of being told I needed surgery, my results are amazing without it. I'm finally able to smile in holiday photos."

—MICHAEL R.

FAQ

Here is a handy resource guide of frequently asked questions and orthodontic terminology, many of which are answered throughout the book.

What might happen if your child's mouth doesn't quite "fit"?

The fact is, the sooner you straighten your child's smile, the faster it will develop as it should: straight, clean, and healthy!

Are there any celebrities who've worn braces?

Many! Gwen Stefani, Prince Harry, Drew Barrymore, Tom Cruise, Dakota Fanning, Danny Glover, and more.

Can I see what my child's straight teeth might look like before the procedure is done?

Yes! Digital pictures are often used to portray what the child's teeth might look like once the braces have been removed.

Will I be able to afford my child's braces?

Not only are most orthodontic procedures cheaper than ever, but insurance, payment plans, and a variety of other financing options make braces more affordable than they've ever been.

Will getting braces be painful for my child?

Not anymore! Modern technology—and choosing the right orthodontist—can ensure that your child enjoys a pain-free orthodontic experience.

How much school will my child miss because of braces?

Not much, actually. After initial visits and, barring the actual procedure itself, most visits and/or adjustments are routine and can take anywhere from fifteen to forty-five minutes.

Is it really such a big deal if my child has crooked teeth?

Unfortunately, yes. Eroding, crooked, or unaligned smiles can take time to happen, but the time to act is now. Orthodontic irregularities don't just heal on their own or "go away" if you ignore them.

What are some of the warning signs that my child might need to go to the orthodontist?

There are many, but here are a few of the most common: early or late loss of teeth, protruding teeth, grinding or clenching of teeth, and speech difficulty.

What kind of "side effects" are caused by crooked teeth?

Some of the more frequent ones we see include headaches, cavities, gum disease, toothaches, mouth breathing, chipped or worn down teeth, snoring, and drooling.

What makes an orthodontist more qualified than a dentist?

Orthodontists are *dental specialists* who have completed two to three years of additional education beyond dental school to learn the proper way to align teeth and jaws.

Why should I choose a specialist for my child's orthodontic care?

Unique treatment requirements and otherwise difficult bite problems are common, everyday scenarios for your orthodontist. In the interest of receiving the most efficient and effective orthodontic treatment possible, choose an orthodontic specialist.

How do I know if my doctor is an orthodontist?

Only orthodontists can belong to the American Association of Orthodontists (AAO).

What is a treatment coordinator?

During your initial consultation(s), you will usually be assigned a patient contact person—we call this person a "treatment coordinator" in our office. This person will help you with your initial orthodontic consultation appointment, help to get you started in braces, help you with scheduling appointments and, of course, answer any and all questions you may have.

Why are follow-up visits important?

These are wonderful opportunities to either a) ask questions you may have missed the first time, or b) get further details from your orthodontist him- or herself.

Why is early evaluation/treatment so important?

Age seven is the earliest time your orthodontist can determine future jaw and tooth alignment. That's because, at the age of seven, your child's upper and lower permanent front teeth are developing. These teeth set the stage for future jaw position and serious problems can develop if they come into the wrong position.

Is there such a thing as a child being too old for braces?

Short answer, no. However, there are definite advantages to bringing your child in for a consultation before they turn ten. We discuss the benefits of this and the risk of waiting until they're in their teens in chapter 1.

What if I don't believe in early orthodontics?

Well, you're entitled to your opinion, but this is like saying you don't believe in the sun. You can hide from it, pretend it's not there, or refuse to acknowledge it, but the simple fact remains. If you're not aware of the potential risks, you can get burnt.

Will my child actually need braces at seven?

Probably not. While we inform parents their child needs an initial exam at age seven, we also mention that most children *will not need braces until eleven to thirteen years of age.*

What is a crossbite?

When the upper and lower teeth grow at different rates, or even when the lower jaw grows disproportionately with the upper jaw, something known as a "crossbite" can occur.

Where should I start to look for treatment if I'm concerned about my child's jaw development?

If you suspect your child might have a crossbite or other issues, approach your family dentist and ask about orthodontics.

Why should I address a crossbite?

Crossbites can lead to pain, discomfort, and lack of confidence as your child begins to feel insecure or even ostracized because of this very treatable, very normal series of jaw and teeth developments.

What is Invisalign?

The Invisalign system is the virtually invisible way to straighten your teeth and achieve the dazzling smile you've always dreamed of. Using advanced 3-D computer-imaging technology, Invisalign depicts your complete treatment plan, from the initial position of your teeth to the final desired position.

What are the primary benefits of Invisalign?

Like the word that inspired them, Invisalign aligners are practically clear and as close to "invisible" as one can get. No one may even notice you're wearing these virtually invisible braces, making Invisalign a seamless fit with your lifestyle and day-to-day interactions with others.

How do I get started with Invisalign?

It's simple: just make an appointment with your local orthodontist for an initial consultation. Most doctors will offer a free initial consultation to see if you are a good candidate for Invisalign.

How will Invisalign effectively move my teeth?

Aligners are the foundation for, and work in unison with, the Invisalign system. Like brackets and arch wires are to braces, Invisalign aligners move teeth by using the appropriate placement of controlled force on your child's teeth.

How many patients are being treated with Invisalign?

More than one million patients worldwide have been treated with Invisalign. The number of Invisalign smiles grows daily.

Is Invisalign appropriate for my child?

Yes, especially because Invisalign now has a system designed specifically for teens!

How does Invisalign Teen work?

Aligners snap on your teeth easily. They are comfortable and practically invisible. Invisalign Teen allows permanent teeth to grow and gently and continuously moves your teeth in small increments. Aligners are worn for about two weeks, then you swap them for a new pair.

Why are metal braces still so popular?

Metal braces are very strong and can withstand most types of treatment. Today's metal braces are smaller, sleeker, and more popular than ever before.

Are so-called "clear braces" effective?

Ceramic braces are very strong and generally do not stain. Adults like to choose ceramic braces because they "blend in" with the teeth and are less noticeable than metal. These are the types of braces actor Tom Cruise had.

Are clear braces appropriate for adults?

Absolutely! Adults of all ages can enjoy the same cosmetic and health benefits of properly aligned teeth with the In-Ovation C system and Radiance braces.

What are some of my payment options in addition to insurance?

Our office is the leader in making orthodontic treatment affordable with no down payment and low monthly payments. Please see the full description of this program in chapter 8. Another way many patients pay for their braces is by utilizing the benefits of what is known as "flex spending," where their employer matches their spending commitment.

What if my child has a "braces emergency" before or after office hours?

If you are experiencing an orthodontic emergency that can't wait for regular office hours, most orthodontic offices have a special number to call, either before, during, or after business hours. If this information isn't given to you readily, ask how your doctor's office handles emergencies.

Can a salt water rinse help deal with irritation caused by braces?

Absolutely; warm saltwater rinses soothe the cheek lining, which can get aggravated by your child's braces.

How do I make a salt water rinse?

To make a salt water rinse, mix half a teaspoon of table salt in one cup of warm water. Stir until the salt is completely dissolved. Gently swish about a fourth of the cup in your mouth for thirty seconds. Make sure you force the water over the areas that feel sore. Then spit the water into the sink. Repeat until the entire cup is gone.

What if my child plays sports and needs a mouth guard?

The best advice for patients or parents looking for a mouth guard can be obtained from your pediatrician, dentist, pediatric dentist, orthodontist or oral surgeon. All of these specialists are uniquely trained to offer customized advice in order to help you prevent a sports-related dental or facial injury.

What about brushing with braces?

Here are some simple tips you can share with your child for the best results when brushing with braces on:

- Brush your teeth with a soft or medium nylon toothbrush after you eat and before bed.

- Brush, rinse, and look; if you find any areas that are not clean, brush them again.

- Brush your gums as you brush your teeth (massage and stimulate).

- If no toothpaste is available, brush without.

- If you are unable to brush, rinse your mouth vigorously with water.

- Replace your old toothbrush when it gets worn out.

- It is absolutely essential that you continue regular visits to your family dentist for checkups and cleanings throughout your orthodontic treatment!

What type of foods should my child avoid while wearing braces?

There are four main types of food your child should avoid while wearing braces: (1) **hard foods**, like ice, popcorn, peanut brittle, rock candy, and corn on the cob, (2) **sticky foods**, like caramels, bubble gum, taffy, and suckers, (3) **chewy foods**, like pizza crust, crusty breads, beef jerky, and gummy bears, and (4) **sugary foods and drinks**, like cake, ice cream, cookies, pie, candy, and soda pop.

Why are retainers so important?

As we age, teeth naturally shift to the middle and crowd. Combined with late growth of the lower jaw, shifting of the teeth is expected following orthodontic treatment. Therefore, retainers are extremely important in the maintenance of your new smile following orthodontic treatment.

Resources

Before or after your consultation, you may want more information for yourself or your son or daughter. The following websites provide valuable insight to help you make the right decision for your child.

Braces.org is the "all about braces site" of the American Association of Orthodontists. This is the official regulatory body and professional association of orthodontists, and *only* orthodontists (*not* dentists) can be members. Here you will receive accurate, up-to-date information on orthodontics.

ExcellenceInOrthodontics.org is the elite association of orthodontists subscribing to a pledge of clinical and customer services excellence. A complete collection of information for patients and parents can be found here.

About the Authors

Michael F. McCarthy, DMD, received his orthodontic training while serving in the military. During his ten years in the US Army, Dr. McCarthy rose to the rank of Major and served as a Green Beret. He is a board-certified orthodontist with over twenty-five years of experience and has been recognized as one of America's Top Dentist by the Consumer Research Council of America every year for the past decade.

Erika Hartman, DDS, was inducted into Omicron Kappa Upsilon dental honor society while at Meharry Medical College and received several honors there, including the Academy of Operative Dentistry student award and the American Association of Orthodontists student award. She received the Faculty Award in Orthodontics while at Howard University for having the highest academic average in her post-graduate orthodontic class. In 2017, Dr. Hartman was recognized as one of America's Top Dentist by the Consumer Research Council of America. She is a member of the American Association of Orthodontists.

Careybeth Rivers, DMD, MS, is a member of the Phi Beta Kappa and Phi Kappa Phi honor societies, and finished second in her class at The University of Alabama, Birmingham, where she received honors such as Omicron Kappa Upsilon, the Leon H. Schneyer award, and the Hinman Scholar award. Upon graduation, she completed an advanced education in general dentistry at the Veterans Administration Hospital in Birmingham where she treated some of the most complex dental cases. She remains active in her church and community, and currently serves on the Make-A-Wish Advisory Council.

THE
NEXT
STEP

Your Customized Smile Analysis

When you are ready, I urge you to schedule your Customized Smile Analysis, complete with a complimentary consultation, safe, digital x-rays (a $249 value) an exam, and a report provided to you and your son or daughter—all without cost or obligation.

> Call us at **205-733-2022** or go to **bhamorthodontics.com**.

Printed in the USA
CPSIA information can be obtained
at www.ICGtesting.com
JSHW012036140824
68134JS00033B/3100

9 781642 250305